Every Woman's Guide to Breast Cancer

Prevention, Treatment, Recovery

Vicki L. Seltzer, M.D.

EVERY WOMAN'S GUIDE TO BREAST CANCER

PREVENTION, TREATMENT, RECOVERY

VIKING

VIKING
Viking Penguin Inc., 40 West 23rd Street,
New York, New York 10010, U.S.A.
Penguin Books Ltd, Harmondsworth,
Middlesex, England
Penguin Books Australia Ltd, Ringwood,
Victoria, Australia
Penguin Books Canada Limited, 2801 John Street,
Markham, Ontario, Canada L3R 1B4
Penguin Books (N.Z.) Ltd, 182–190 Wairau Road,
Auckland 10, New Zealand

First published in 1987 by Viking Penguin Inc.
Published simultaneously in Canada

LIBRARY OF CONGRESS CATALOGING IN PUBLICATION DATA
Seltzer, Vicki L.
Every woman's guide to breast cancer.
1. Breast—Cancer—Popular works.   I. Title.
[DNLM: 1. Breast Neoplasms—popular works.
WP 870 S468e]
RC280.B8S44   1987   616.99′449   86-40495
ISBN 0-670-80923-3

Printed in the United States of America by
R. R. Donnelley & Sons Company, Harrisonburg, Virginia
Set in Bembo

To Richard, Herb, Marian, Jessica, and Eric
Thank you for your love, patience, and support

Acknowledgments

This manuscript was written over a period of several years, and it could not have been completed without the assistance of many dear friends and colleagues. Most significantly, my husband, Richard Brach, was an enormous source of encouragement and support, as he has been in every facet of my life. I also wish to thank my parents, and Jessica and Eric, constant sources of inspiration.

Several of my medical colleagues have been most helpful. I have received advice from many physicians with whom I have worked in the past, who provide dedicated, sensitive medical care to women suffering from malignancies. I would like to thank Dr. Herschel Flax for his guidance and for the photographs of women whom he has treated for breast cancer by lumpectomy and radiation therapy. He is a fine, innovative surgeon and was an early supporter of conservative surgery for breast cancer. I thank Dr. Frederick Lukash for the photographs of the beautiful, artistic surgery that he has performed for breast reconstruction. I also want to thank three excellent chemotherapists, both for their guidance with this book and for their very fine care of my patients during the past several years: Dr. Steven Vogl, Dr. Marc Citron, and Dr. Jagmamohan Kalra. Two radiation therapists, early supporters of radiation therapy as primary treatment for breast cancer, have been of great assistance in the preparation of this manuscript: Dr. André Abitbol and Dr. Jay Cooper. Dr. Martin Tindell, who has dedicated much of his career to the surgical therapy of patients with malignancy, has also been a great help.

I would like to thank Dr. Fred Benjamin and Dr. Joseph J. Rovinsky for their constant support and encouragement. Thanks also to those physicians—very fine doctors and teachers—who helped me to acquire my medical skills and also an understanding of the multifaceted needs of patients with malignancy: Dr. John L. Lewis, Jr., Dr. Walter Jones, Dr. Sanford Sall, Dr. Antonio Calanog, Dr. Martin L. Stone, Dr. Gordon Watkins Douglas, Dr. Robert Porges, Dr. Stan Zinberg, Dr. Bruce Young, Dr. E. Mark Beckman, Dr. Harold Shulman, and Dr. Lila Wallis.

Knowing all that I know about being a physician, I still could not have written this book without the guidance of Caroline Bird, a very fine author and a dear friend. Other friends who were most generous with their guidance and support include Dr. Helen DeRosis, Karen W. Arenson, Dulcina Eisen, Mel Berger, and Ken Norwick. Maria McNally has been of great assistance, always patient, always positive, always helpful. I would especially like to thank Dawn Seferian. She has worked so energetically with me, and has been constantly supportive and encouraging. And I appreciate Constance Sayre and Kathryn Court for realizing how important this book can be for women, and how much it can do to improve their health.

Last of all, I would like to thank my patients. It gives me such pleasure to help people to be healthier and to feel better about their lives.

This book was written to teach women about their bodies, to prevent unnecessary physical and psychological pain, and to help prevent completely avoidable deaths. It should help women to ask the right questions so that they can effectively participate in decisions regarding their health care and be in greater control of their futures. However, it is essential to remember that every patient and medical problem is unique and that only a physician who has examined you personally and is fully aware of the details of your particular condition can be able to render an appropriate medical opinion.

There are many differences of opinion in the medical literature regarding almost every aspect of breast cancer. In addition, new data are coming to our attention almost daily. I have tried to present a balanced view of all the issues, many of which do not have conclusive answers.

This book is not intended to, and cannot, provide you with a specific medical opinion that applies directly to your particular situation. For every issue relating to breast cancer, from the frequency of screening to the diagnosis and treatment of disease, you must obtain the opinion of one or more physicians who know your specific history and have examined you.

The case histories in this book do not describe the stories of individual women. Rather, they represent situations that commonly occur.

Contents

Contents

Contents

CHAPTER I

An Open Letter
to Women

To all women over the age of twenty,

I am concerned about you and I have written this book
because breast cancer is a disease that is approaching epidemic proportions, and we women must take appropriate
measures to safeguard ourselves. One of every eleven
women born in the United States today will develop breast
cancer. There is a great deal that we can be doing to improve our odds, yet during more than a decade of providing health care for women, I have noticed that so many
patients are reluctant to participate in an appropriate program of prevention and screening. I have written this book
to tell you how much you can do for yourselves. This book
can save your life.

Some information available at present suggests that there
are ways to reduce the risk of developing breast cancer,
and, perhaps, even to prevent it for some women. Certainly the prevention of the disease is our ultimate goal.

This book will explain to you what an appropriate
screening program is, and how you may properly participate. It will explain how important it is to have your physician involved in your screening program, and will tell

you which warning signals make it imperative for you to consult your doctor immediately.

If breast cancer is detected early, the tumor can usually be cured, frequently without the removal of the breast. This is done by removing the cancer and a small amount of normal surrounding tissue, removing lymph nodes in the underarm, and treating the cancer with radiation. The cosmetic results are usually excellent, and it is common for the breast that previously harbored the malignancy to look the same as the normal breast. On the other hand, when breast cancer is detected in a more advanced state, the chances for cure diminish significantly, and the required surgery will more likely have to include removal of the breast, which often causes considerable psychological as well as physical trauma.

The probability of developing breast cancer is significantly greater than that of being involved in an airplane accident. However, every time we board an airplane, the flight attendants provide us with a lengthy explanation and a visual demonstration of how to proceed in case of an emergency. Since people tend to panic in crisis situations, the appropriate disaster procedures are discussed during the calm minutes surrounding the takeoff.

When people learn that they have cancer, the reaction is frequently and understandably one of panic. This is true not only with cancer of the breast, but with all malignancies. Since breast cancer occurs with such great frequency, and since this particular type of malignancy arouses such great emotional impact, the wise woman will inform herself about the disease while she is healthy. All women should learn about the various forms of therapy, especially about the pros and cons of preserving the breast. Although every situation is different, and only a doctor who has examined you can make recommendations for your individual care, several different therapeutic options may be appropriate for any one patient's breast cancer. It is inordinately difficult to assimilate all this information and make a decision within a period of several days once the disease has been diagnosed.

I hope that you will never need this information for yourself. But if you have just six friends, there is a reasonable possibility that one or more has had or will develop breast cancer. What you will learn in this book may ultimately be invaluable to you in coming to the aid of a friend.

There is another way in which this book can save lives—the lives of your friends, and maybe your own. Women with breast cancer that has advanced to involve the lymph nodes have less than a forty-percent chance of living for ten years. On the other hand, women whose breast malignancy has been diagnosed early may have better than a seventy-percent chance of avoiding a recurrence during the next ten years. Early diagnosis saves lives; this book will help you learn how the diagnosis can be made promptly.

Many women are uncomfortable with the idea of self-examination and screening for early breast cancer: "Why look for trouble?" they ask. I call it the "can't happen to me" syndrome, because everyone believes that this problem will only happen to someone else. Unfortunately, it can happen to any one of us.

I am hoping that most of the women who read this book will be healthy. Much of what I've written is about how to stay healthy—addressing such issues as how to reduce your risk of developing a breast malignancy and how to become involved in a proper screening program.

However, this book will also be of great value for the woman who has already been treated for breast cancer. If you have had the disease, it will help you to become more comfortable and knowledgeable about the future, and encourage you to continue to enjoy your life. It will provide guidance for both the physical and the emotional aspects of coping with the disease, considering such topics as breast reconstruction, sexuality after mastectomy, the psychological impact of breast cancer, and additional medical therapy (radiation, chemotherapy, hormones). I also discuss the importance of appropriate follow-up and what you can expect following the initial therapy.

I have written this book because I feel that we women are not doing enough to help ourselves. The advice that I give is simple and straightforward, and based upon more than a decade of experience in providing health care for women.

As a doctor and as a woman, I am overwhelmingly saddened to see lives needlessly lost, and to treat women who have suffered because of their inattention to their own bodies. My greatest wish for you all is that you will not be the one in eleven who will be affected. But the risk is extraordinarily high, and it cannot be ignored.

Please read this book and follow its very simple advice. Then give it to someone you love.

Sincerely,

Vicki L. Seltzer, md

Vicki L. Seltzer, M.D.

CHAPTER II

The Magnitude
of the Problem

Among all American women who die when they are
between the ages of forty and forty-five, the cause of death
most likely to be listed on the death certificate is BREAST
CANCER. Breast and lung tumors are responsible for the
greatest number of deaths due to malignancy among
American women, and breast cancer alone is the cause of
almost one-fifth of all cancer-related mortalities in women.
It results in approximately thirty-seven thousand deaths
annually in the United States alone. Each year the disease
is diagnosed in more than one hundred thousand American
women and several times that number worldwide.

Unfortunately, we do not yet have control of this pub-
lic-health problem, a problem that in many ways is beginning to reach epidemic proportions. In fact, the incidence
of breast cancer is continuing to increase rather than decreasing. And there is no time in a woman's life when she
can rest assured that she is no longer at risk, since the likelihood of developing breast malignancies continues to increase as a woman ages. Breast cancer is a disease that begins
to strike women when they are in the prime of their lives,
then goes on to be a relentless adversary. The disease commonly affects women in their forties, but if a woman passes

through that decade in good health, she is at even greater risk in her fifties. Indeed, through each decade in which a woman passes unharmed, her potential for developing breast cancer continues to increase.

The questions we must ask ourselves are: Can anything be done to decrease the mortality from this disease? Can we work effectively to make the incidence of this malignancy start to decline rather than keep increasing? Can a woman reduce her own risk, either of developing breast cancer or of dying from this malignancy?

The answer to each of these questions is yes. As you continue to read, you will see how preventive techniques can enable you as an individual, and us as a society, to diminish the potential for developing breast cancer. You will learn how, individually and collectively, we can reduce, for those unfortunate women who are afflicted, the likelihood of their dying from breast cancer.

Not only is the risk to any American woman of developing breast cancer inordinately high, but certain features place some women at even greater risk than others. Some of these risk factors, either singly or in aggregate, raise a woman's chance of developing breast cancer to well over fifteen percent. It is important to consider these factors carefully, since some of them are environmental, and a highly motivated woman may decide to modify a few aspects of her life style to lessen the probability of developing breast cancer.

One of the major factors placing a woman at risk is a family history of the disease. Approximately one-quarter of all American women with breast cancer have had a family member who has been afflicted with it. Having a mother or a sister with breast cancer causes a greater increase in the risk than any other component of the family history, and if the sister is a twin the potential for developing a malignancy is still greater. In addition, if a woman's mother had breast cancer before entering menopause, or if she had cancer in both breasts, then her daughter's chances of developing the disease are even greater.

Having other relatives (for instance, grandmothers or aunts) who have had breast cancer will also increase a woman's risk, and having female relatives in more than one generation afflicted with the disease probably further increases it. Breast cancer is likely to strike women in succeeding generations approximately ten years earlier than it did those in the first generation affected.

If you have had a family member with breast cancer, you must regard yourself as at greater risk than the average woman (and, after all, we are really all at high risk of developing the disease just by virtue of being women). I encourage women with family members who have had breast cancer even more strongly than the already emphatic advice that I give to the average woman, to participate in a screening program for breast cancer. This should include monthly breast self-examination, frequent physical examination by a doctor (for very high-risk women this may be recommended as often as every six months until age thirty-five, and every three months thereafter), and a regular program of screening mammography (as outlined in a later chapter).

Often a woman whose mother or sister or other close relative had breast cancer will be frightened by the thought of a tumor. She may have helped her relative through periods of physical or emotional trauma, and possibly be scarred by this herself. In an attempt to forget the pain her loved one experienced, the relative of the breast-cancer patient may try to avoid the issue entirely by purposely not using breast-cancer screening, even though she fully understands how important it is. Unfortunately, this is exactly the type of woman for whom screening is so significant.

Shirley Parkerson, an attractive forty-five-year-old college English professor who was married but had no children, brought her sixty-eight-year-old mother, Janet McClain, to the doctor's office. Mrs. Parkerson told the doctor that she was very upset with her mother because Mrs. McClain had had breast cancer seven years earlier but had been delinquent in maintaining her follow-up appointments. Mrs. McClain had had a mastectomy, and was depressed for about six months following the surgery. Whereas she had been quite meticulous about having regular checkups before the mastectomy—indeed, it was during an annual examination that her physician had detected her cancer—she had rarely seen the doctor since her surgery. Although following surgery the doctor had told her how frequently she must be examined, what follow-up studies would need to be done, and how to perform breast self-examination, Mrs. McClain was not carrying out any of these instructions.

Mrs. Parkerson went on to say that, although she and her mother had always had a wonderful relationship before her mother got breast cancer, and she had helped her mother both physically and psychologically during the months after surgery, the two had been fighting a lot during the last several years, often about Mrs. Parkerson's anger that her mother was not continuing with her follow-up appointments.

The doctor examined Mrs. McClain and found her to be in good health. He then explained in detail to both women the program he was recommending for Mrs. McClain (including self-examination, physician appointments, and X-ray and blood studies).

As he was completing the consultation, he casually mentioned to Mrs. Parkerson that he assumed she was performing monthly self-examination, being examined regularly by her physician, and having screening mammography. He was astonished to discover that Mrs. Parkerson was not doing anything at all to be screened for breast disease. The doctor urged her to see her own physician and to get actively involved in a screening program.

Three months later, Mrs. Parkerson called her mother's doctor to make an appointment for herself. She revealed to him that she had never performed self-examination, never had a mammography, and rarely saw a doctor at all. Upon further questioning, she admitted that ever since her mother's mastectomy she had been extremely fearful that she, too, would develop breast cancer. However, instead of approaching this fear head-on and taking care of herself properly, she avoided the issue. Although she realized this was a completely irrational response to her anxiety, taking care of her mother had rendered her incapable of dealing with her own potential for the illness.

The doctor explained to her at length that the statistics were real and would not go away. She had a very significant risk of developing breast cancer, both because her mother had had the disease and because she had had no children. This risk might possibly be diminished by careful attention to diet, but it would never be low. However, if she did develop breast cancer but was being properly and regularly screened, so that the illness could be discovered in its earliest phase, she would have an excellent chance of being cured. In addition, cure could probably be achieved by removal of the lump and radiation, without requiring the removal of her breast. With counseling, Mrs. Parkerson was able to accept the fact that, even if avoidance of the issue temporarily relieved her anxiety, true peace of mind would come only with regular breast self-examination and a careful screening program.

In addition to family history, another factor that significantly alters a woman's risk of developing breast cancer is her reproductive history. A woman with no children has almost one and a half times as much chance of developing breast cancer as does a woman who has children. The age of a woman when her first child is born is also significant. A woman who has her first child before she is twenty diminishes her risk by one-half. Some data suggest that a woman who waits until she is in her mid- to late thirties or older to have her first child will be under even greater risk than will a woman without children. Clearly, the childbearing practices of our society have changed during the past few decades. Large numbers of women have decided to defer pregnancy until they are much older, or not to have children at all, for reasons intertwined with advances in career opportunities and a system of values and personal goals that is considerably different from that which existed two decades ago. Since this trend may well be permanent, the risk of breast cancer for our population could continue to increase.

Someone who has had cancer in one breast is at extremely high risk of developing a new primary cancer (in other words, a completely new tumor; not a metastasis—spread—from the previous tumor) in the other breast. This is even more likely to happen if the woman's first malignancy occurred before she entered menopause. Such women occasionally elect to undergo a prophylactic removal of the tissue of the other breast (removal of a breast that is, at the time, completely normal and disease-free), a practice that is extremely controversial. Since breast cancer can usually be diagnosed early in its course if a woman is properly screened, and since a woman doesn't necessarily have to lose her breast at all even if she does develop a malignancy, many people feel that the removal of a normal breast merely for preventive purposes is unnecessarily extreme. However, some women feel that if they have had cancer in one breast, the constant fear of developing another cancer in the other breast is reason enough. The decision is an extremely personal matter, and one that obviously requires very careful consideration. Clearly, in a matter such as this, only the individual, who has mulled over both the medical data and her own personal needs, can determine what is correct for her.

Many doctors believe that women who have *true* fibrocystic disease are at increased risk of developing breast cancer. However, "fibrocystic disease" is an overdiagnosed problem; indeed, two physicians examining the same breast might disagree as to whether it deserves the label. Since there is a lot of controversy regarding the disease entity itself, it is difficult to calculate the risk for breast cancer that the presence of fibrocystic disease would present. So many women have been told that they have fibrocystic disease, and are quite appropriately concerned about whether more serious problems may occur as a result of this, that I have devoted a later chapter exclusively to this problem.

Prolonged menstrual activity, due either to an early onset of menstruation or to a late menopause, will increase a woman's risk of developing breast cancer. During the years in which a woman has menstrual periods, the volume of hormones produced by her ovaries is greatly increased. These hormones, which are made by her own body, may increase her breast-cancer risk. A woman who began to menstruate before her twelfth birthday may have as much as twice the risk of developing breast cancer as a woman who began having her periods when she was thirteen or older. If a woman's menstrual periods end naturally before she is forty-five years of age, she has half the risk of developing breast cancer that someone who reaches menopause when she is fifty-five or older has. A woman who undergoes a hysterectomy (removal of the uterus) but has her ovaries left in is not protected from breast cancer. However, a woman who has had her ovaries removed before she reaches the age of thirty-five diminishes her risk of developing breast cancer to one-quarter of what would otherwise be expected. All these findings relating to the correlation between menstrual activity and breast tumors strongly suggest that the hormones produced by a woman's own ovaries may play a significant role in affecting her risk of developing breast cancer.

Many women who are going through menopause wish to take estrogen pills. This medication will alleviate hot flashes and prevent osteoporosis (a loss of minerals in the bones, which will increase a woman's risk of fractures). Estrogen will also reduce vaginal dryness (a common problem for women who have gone through menopause, and one that may substantially interfere with sexual interest and comfort during intercourse) and produce other beneficial results. In addition to all these very positive functions, however, estrogen can also cause a few undesirable side effects. Since the body's own hormones appear to have some potential role in affecting a woman's risk of developing breast cancer, there was great concern about whether one of the negative effects of estrogen pills would be to increase the risk of breast cancer. In April 1983, the Centers for Disease Control in Atlanta reported that a woman who takes estrogen for menopausal symptomatology does not appear to increase her chances of developing breast cancer. This information, based upon extensive research, brought a sense of relief to many women.

On the other hand, some physicians are wary of prescribing estrogen for women who have other high-risk factors, such as a family history of breast cancer. These doctors are concerned that, even if estrogen does not appear to cause breast problems for women who do not have high-risk factors, it might have a greater likelihood of causing breast problems in high-risk women.

Under almost no circumstances would a physician prescribe estrogen to ease menopausal symptomatology for a woman who has already had breast cancer: it has been established that once such a tumor is present, estrogen may result in rapid worsening of the disease. Even if a woman has completed therapy for breast cancer, the use of estrogen may precipitate a more rapid recurrence of the malignancy.

Oral contraceptives are used widely in the United States and throughout the world. Most women who use the pill feel that its benefits for them outweigh its risks and that it has afforded them the opportunity to plan their families and their lives. All women who use the birth-control pill know that it has potential risks. Since it contains estrogen, there has been concern about whether it might affect a woman's risk of developing breast cancer. A few years ago, a report suggested that the use of oral contraceptives could increase this risk. There have been subsequent papers that conclude that birth-control pills do not increase breast-cancer risk. In addition, there *is* evidence that oral contraceptives will decrease a woman's risk of developing ovarian cancer, benign breast disease, fibrocystic breast disease, and serious pelvic infection. Most doctors, at present, feel that there is no proof that the use of birth-control pills will increase a woman's chance of developing breast cancer. Some feel that the problem requires further study before patients can be properly and definitively advised. Doctors are, in general, much less comfortable prescribing the pill for a woman who is in her forties, but this has much more to do with the potential for serious heart problems that birth-control pills may cause in women during their later reproductive years.

A woman who has previously had a cancer of the uterus or of the ovary is also more likely to develop a new primary cancer of the breast. These breast tumors must be sought and treated aggressively: many women have had two unrelated malignancies and been cured of both.

Another very important risk factor is age. As a woman ages, her chances of developing breast cancer increase. Therefore, a woman should never feel that she has "outgrown" the risk and stop examining her breasts. Her susceptibility to the disease at age eighty is even greater than it was when she was fifty.

Obesity appears to increase the likelihood that a postmenopausal woman will develop breast cancer, but this risk factor is one that can be controlled. Overweight women should be advised to follow an appropriate program of weight reduction, not only to help reduce their risk of developing breast cancer. Weight reduction is also important for those women since obesity also increases the likelihood that a woman will develop a vast range of other life-threatening conditions, including high blood pressure, heart disease, diabetes, and uterine cancer.

Another factor is a woman's socioeconomic status: women in the upper socioeconomic groups are statistically at greater risk of developing breast cancer. The disease also has a racial predilection: Caucasian women are at highest risk for breast cancer, but the disease is now manifesting a tremendous increase in incidence among American black women, who traditionally were at low risk. It is hypothesized that this increase may be related to recent changes in diet and life styles.

Women who live in the Western Hemisphere and in a cold climate are at increased risk. The probability that a woman will have this malignancy is six times higher if she resides in the United States or Canada than if she lives in Asia. But when groups of Japanese women have moved to the United States, their daughters' risk of developing breast cancer begins to increase toward the incidence of breast cancer noted in American women. This is believed to be attributable to environmental influences, particularly to diet: the second-generation Japanese woman often begins to adopt a diet similar to that of the typical American woman, with its very high fat content.

In addition to the aforementioned clinical high-risk factors, there are certain medical observations, made either by machine or by tissue biopsy, that indicate that a woman is at high risk of developing breast cancer. If one of these findings is present in a woman, her doctor can then advise her of what it may mean.

For instance, a mammography, besides demonstrating a specific area of malignancy, can also yield other types of information that may be extremely useful for the patient and her doctor. When radiologists (doctors whose specialty is to interpret X-rays) study a mammography, besides looking for a cancer they are also evaluating the tissue pattern of the breast (called "parenchymal mammographic patterns"). Certain patterns are thought to be associated with a higher risk of developing breast cancer. The radiologist will often provide the patient's personal physician with this information. Then the doctor can use it, along with other facts about the woman, to advise her in planning an appropriate screening program.

Thermograms (discussed extensively in the next chapter) are evaluations of breast tissue based upon the amount of blood flow and heat in each area of the breast. Although they are not as accurate in diagnosing malignancy as mammograms are, patients whose thermograms are abnormal but in whom no malignancy has been demonstrated have been noted to have a higher risk of eventually developing breast cancer. Therefore, if a woman has an abnormal thermogram but breast cancer is not detected, her doctor will advise her to be followed very closely.

Certain findings from a breast biopsy may also indicate that a woman is at increased risk. When someone has a breast biopsy, the first question she naturally asks is "Was it malignant?" Every ounce of energy and attention is usually focused on this one very important question. The relief, even elation, is overwhelming when a woman hears that the biopsy did not show malignancy. However, there are some findings on biopsy that, while not truly malignant, do indicate that the woman is at increased risk to develop a malignancy. One such finding is the biopsy report of lobular carcinoma *in situ*, a premalignant lesion. Approximately one-quarter of women who are found on breast biopsy to have lobular carcinoma *in situ* will ultimately develop a true invasive (malignant) breast cancer. The malignancy may appear either in the breast that had been affected with carcinoma *in situ* or in the other breast.

There are other findings that may be discovered at the time of a breast biopsy that are not malignant, and do not carry so high a risk of subsequent breast cancer as does lobular carcinoma *in situ*, but that do indicate that a woman is at increased risk. Whereas carcinoma *in situ* may sometimes be treated by mastectomy, these other findings are often managed by careful observation, once the possibility of cancer has been eliminated and any necessary diagnostic or therapeutic surgery completed. An example of this is fibrocystic disease.

Two steps must be taken in the evaluation of high-risk factors, depending on whether a given factor can or cannot be altered. First, and most important, a woman should be made aware of which specific features of her family history or her life style place her at high risk of developing breast cancer. She should then evaluate these high-risk features in terms of her present life, and identify those factors that can be eliminated and those that cannot be altered.

The high-risk factors that can readily be eliminated from a woman's life include obesity and a dietary intake high in fat. By controlling these, a woman can also decrease her risk for developing a wide variety of other medical disorders.

Some factors cannot be altered. A woman cannot change the fact that her mother and sister have had breast cancer, for instance. But if she is aware that her family history places her at exceedingly high risk for the disease, she can participate in an aggressive screening program.

Once a woman fully understands the risk factors, that knowledge becomes power. She can alter some of the risk factors, and perhaps prevent herself from ever becoming afflicted with breast cancer. Of, if the risks are unalterable, she can participate conscientiously in a breast-cancer detection program so that if she does develop the disease it can be diagnosed early, while it is curable, and more likely curable without requiring the removal of her breast.

CHAPTER III

Screening Techniques

It is the rule with most malignancies that the earlier the disease is diagnosed, the greater is the likelihood that the patient can be cured. This is certainly true of breast cancer. If a breast cancer is diagnosed when it is less than half a centimeter in size (about the size of a small pea), there may be as high as a ninety-five-percent chance that the patient will be alive ten years later. On the other hand, patients with larger masses that have metastasized to the lymph nodes in the underarm may have less than a forty-percent chance of being alive ten years later. It is abundantly clear, therefore, that we must ensure that women are being properly and regularly screened for breast cancer, so that if a tumor develops it will be diagnosed in its earliest phase, before it begins to spread. When we further consider that early breast cancers are frequently curable without requiring mastectomy, it becomes clear how vital screening programs are.

So many women know about the risks of breast cancer and about the various methods of breast-cancer screening, yet only a small proportion of them are involved in any form of screening program. The following is a sample of some of the explanations that I have heard from women rationalizing why they do not participate: "Why look for trouble?" "I couldn't cope with it if I were found to have breast cancer." "What I don't know can't hurt me." "If I am found to have breast cancer, I will have to undergo mutilating surgery."

My responses to these remarks are as follows: For the woman who says "Why look for trouble?" the answer is that, whether or not she looks for it, the trouble may already be there, and that early discovery of the problem significantly diminishes the risks. For the woman who states "I couldn't cope with it if I were found to have breast cancer," the answer is that ultimately she will have to cope. If it is diagnosed early, she will probably have to cope only with treatment of the disease. If it is found late, she is more likely to have to cope with the prospect of dying as a result of the malignancy. The choice, therefore, may be to cope sooner with a significant problem or to cope later with a situation of much more enormous magnitude. To the woman who says "What I don't know can't hurt me," I say that, unfortunately, it may not just hurt her but ultimately kill her. To the woman whose rationale is "If I am found to have breast cancer, I will have to undergo mutilating surgery," I explain the paradox that if she participates in a screening program and the breast cancer is diagnosed sufficiently early, she has the greatest opportunity to be cured without having to have a mastectomy.

Clearly, screening programs for breast cancer should be used by all women, with guidance from their doctors. Screening programs can certainly save lives, and they can, in addition, greatly improve the odds for a good cosmetic outcome.

Although a significant component of a screening program involves instrumentation (mammography), this is only one part of a three-pronged approach to the early detection of breast cancer. The screening triad, each component of which is extremely important, includes self-examination, examination by a physician, and radiologic screening by mammography.

The American Cancer Society has issued guidelines regarding the early detection of breast cancer in asymptomatic women (women who do not have any known problems). Their recommendations are always being re-evaluated but at the time of this writing are:

1. All women, from the age of twenty on, should perform monthly breast self-examination.

2. Examination of the breast by a doctor should begin at age twenty, should be performed at least once every three years thereafter, and must be done annually once a woman reaches the age of forty.

3. A preliminary mammogram should be performed at some time between the ages of thirty-five and forty. Between the ages of forty and forty-nine, mammography is performed every one to two years. Women over the age of fifty should have annual mammography.

These guidelines are for screening. That means that they are a plan for the regular evaluation of healthy women, so that, should an abnormality occur, it can be found and treated as early as possible. Women who have already had problems with their breasts, or who appear to be at very high risk for developing breast cancer, may be advised to be followed even more frequently. In addition, any woman who notices a problem with her breast should obviously consult her physician immediately.

Breast self-examination, which will be described in detail in the next chapter, is an extremely useful aid in the diagnosis of breast cancer, and should be performed monthly. For a woman who is still menstruating, I recommend to my patients that it be done on the seventh day after her menstrual period begins. For the woman who is no longer menstruating, I recommend that it be performed on the first day of each month. Since most women have a doctor examine their breasts and undergo mammography annually at most, monthly self-examination gives a woman the opportunity to detect an early malignancy that may become apparent in the interval between medical screenings. And since no technology is ever one-hundred-percent accurate, a woman may diagnose by self-examination a breast cancer that was missed by mammography.

Unfortunately, even though breast self-examination costs nothing, is simple to perform, and takes only a few minutes each month, it has been estimated that only one in five women in the United States performs it regularly. This is shocking in such an educated society, in which so much medical and media attention has been given to the issue. I strongly urge you to use the techniques for breast self-examination that I will describe. Do it carefully every month, and encourage all the other women you care about to do the same.

My recommendation for screening by a physician, the program I suggest to my own patients, is even more rigorous than the plan offered by the American Cancer Society. I agree that unless a woman is symptomatic, or discovers a lump during breast self-examination, or notes any breast abnormality, her first breast examination by a doctor does not need to be performed until she is twenty. I recommend to my patients that once they reach the age of thirty-five, however, they should have annual breast examinations by a physician, and if they have significant high-risk factors, such examinations should probably be performed every six months at least.

My recommendation to my patients between the ages of twenty and thirty-five differs somewhat from that of the American Cancer Society. I advise all patients that, once they have begun to have intercourse, they should have a pelvic exam and Pap smear annually, since they now become at risk of developing premalignant (an abnormality that has the potential to develop into a malignancy) and malignant cervical tumors, and the Pap smear will reduce their risk of mortality from cervical cancer. Clearly, when a woman is being seen annually for her pelvic exam and Pap smear, the breast examination can be done with minimal additional time or effort on the part of the patient. So, if a woman between the ages of twenty and thirty-five is being seen annually by a doctor, I feel she should have a breast examination at the time of her visits. On the other hand, if for some reason a woman who is between these ages and in a low-risk group is not having regular medical examinations, even though her risk of breast cancer is small, she should still visit a doctor to have her breasts examined every three years.

Occasionally, a breast examination by a woman herself or by her physician will detect a breast tumor that is not discovered by mammography. This might occur for a few reasons. As mentioned earlier, no single medical test, including mammography, is one-hundred-percent accurate. There are rare instances in which a breast tumor may be present, but not be detected by mammography. In addition, a woman will usually be having screening mammography performed once a year at most, and in some instances a palpable tumor may develop between tests. Women can examine their breasts monthly, but obviously should not be subjected to monthly X-rays. Therefore, women who are being regularly screened by mammography should also examine their own breasts and see their doctors on schedule.

However, mammography is an extremely valuable tool that can save lives. It is the only current means of diagnosing with dependable regularity tumors that are too small to be felt by the woman herself or by her physician. And these small tumors are the ones most likely to be curable.

Since screening programs may significantly diminish the rate of mortality from breast cancer by providing earlier diagnoses, there have been a wide range of technologies investigated as potential screening techniques. These include ultrasonography, thermography, diaphanography, CT scanning, and nuclear magnetic resonance imaging (NMR). Each of these will be discussed below, but it is essential to understand that, at present, only mammography screening programs have been demonstrated to reduce breast-cancer mortality, and most physicians feel that at present mammography is the appropriate technique to use.

MAMMOGRAPHY

Mammography was somewhat controversial a decade ago, but in 1987 is widely accepted as an excellent screening technique to diagnose early nonpalpable breast cancer. During the 1960s, mammography began to be used extensively in the United States. In these early studies, the radiation exposure was significantly higher than with the techniques and equipment that are presently utilized. Moreover, the image quality of the mammographic films and the radiologists' training in mammography have both improved considerably since then, enabling even smaller tumors to be diagnosed. And, again, the smaller the tumor when it is found, the better the chances of cure. Data presented from Thomas Jefferson University Hospital in Philadelphia show that only thirteen percent of patients with breast tumors smaller than two centimeters in size had lymph-node metastases, but more than fifty percent of patients with breast tumors two to three centimeters in size had lymph-node metastases. The presence of lymph-node metastases significantly diminishes the likelihood of cure.

From 1963 through 1968, the Health Insurance Plan of Greater New York evaluated the efficacy of mammography in screening for breast cancer and in saving lives. Women members of this health-maintenance organization who were not known to have breast cancer were given the opportunity to participate in the study. They were randomly assigned to one of two groups. One group had mammography performed each year for the five years of the study. The other group of women did not have mammography, but received regular medical care. The result was that for women over the age of fifty who participated in the study, those who had mammography performed had a forty percent reduction in mortality from breast cancer when compared with those who did not receive any special screening.

More recent data, from the Breast Cancer Detection Demonstration Projects, suggest that mammography screening can probably decrease breast-cancer mortality in women from age thirty-five onward. In their study, more than one-third of the cancers in women under the age of fifty were found by mammography alone. And, as we already know, the detection of these very small tumors, not palpable on physical examination, is extremely important, since breast cancer is most curable at this stage of the disease process.

What exactly happens when a mammography is done? In many instances, the physician sends the woman for X-rays, which are taken by the technician and later read by the radiologist. However, many radiologists feel that, even though the woman has usually been examined recently by her own doctor, the radiologist should also examine her and question her regarding her medical history. So, if the radiology staff asks to re-examine you and wants an extensive medical history, what they are attempting to do is to increase their chances of diagnosing any lesion you may have. Some centers, however, do not conduct physical examinations or take detailed histories; policies vary.

Mammography is most commonly done by taking two X-rays of each breast. Occasionally, more than two X-rays of a single breast will be taken. This does not mean that there has been an error, nor is it a sign that you have a serious abnormality. It may just indicate that the radiologist wishes to see the breast tissue at a slightly different angle or that an additional X-ray is needed to capture the entire tail (tissue in the upper, outer portion) of the breast.

Although not painful, mammography frequently produces a brief, moderate amount of discomfort. Mammography X-rays must be taken while the breast is being compressed, and this squeezing of the breast tissue does produce discomfort for a few moments. The compression, though, is essential. First of all, using this technique creates a more accurate X-ray picture of the breast tissue, and a more accurate picture is more likely to reveal any lesions that are present. Second, the compression reduces the radiation dose to the breast tissue. The technique of mammography has continued to improve, and is presently much more accurate, with markedly diminished radiation exposure.

Most women for whom I recommend mammography ask whether the procedure carries any risks—an appropriate question, one that should be asked about any medical procedure. There could possibly be a small amount of risk associated with the radiation dose to the breast when a mammography is done; it is possible that the radiation itself can increase the risk of malignancy for an extremely small number of women. It is essential, however, to note that the radiation exposure to the breast is minimal, particularly when compared with the techniques used a decade ago—and that the possible ill effects of mammography performed at appropriate intervals are extremely small when compared with the enormous contribution mammography can make in the early detection of breast cancer and thus in saving lives.

At present, with new equipment and technology, the average radiation to the breast glands with a two-view mammography should be under one rad (a measure of absorbed radiation), and is often considerably less than that. To put this dosage into perspective, consider that the average amount of radiation required to treat a tumor is approximately five to ten thousand times the dosage produced by mammography. Of course, it is preferable never to be exposed to any radiation, but in medicine one must always assess the risks and benefits of any practice and determine whether the benefits justify the potential risks, no matter how slight those risks may be. In my opinion, the American Cancer Society guidelines on the appropriate use of mammography, as stated earlier in this chapter, are reasonable, and I believe that the benefits of mammography screening for women at the ages and intervals outlined in their guidelines probably justify the small potential risk. It is certainly conceivable that, as more studies are done and more data are collected, these guidelines will continue to be modified over the years. However, according to the information available in 1987, they are appropriate guidelines to be offered at this time.

Other groups have published guidelines that differ somewhat from those of the American Cancer Society. The American College of Radiology, the American College of Obstetricians and Gynecologists, and the National Cancer Institute all have their own, somewhat differing guidelines. There is no definite answer regarding which set of guidelines is best, and you will have to speak with your doctor to determine the best course for you.

XEROMAMMOGRAPHY

In 1972, the technique of xeromammography was introduced by Dr. John N. Wolfe, a radiologist in Detroit. This technique utilizes the same basic principles as the conventional X-ray mammography, but the films are printed on paper and do not require an X-ray view box to be evaluated. Some physicians advocate xeromammography, others the conventional technique. Those who use conventional X-ray mammography say that it results in less radiation exposure, and therefore has less potential risk. Those who prefer xeromammography say that it is better able to find tumors at the back of the breast, near the rib cage. During the past year, the issue of the radiation dose with xeromammography has received even greater attention. It is possible that this will result in decreased use of this technique.

ULTRASOUND

At present, ultrasound cannot be considered a reliable technique to be used alone in screening for breast cancer. This is unfortunate, since it does not produce any radiation exposure and is therefore currently believed to carry no risk. Ultrasound works by passing sound waves through tissue and it can distinguish the presence of an abnormal mass. It appears, however, that a significant percentage of breast cancers that are nonpalpable but can be identified by mammography will be missed by ultrasound. This, of course, is a major disadvantage, since the aim of a screening technique is to detect tumors as early as possible.

I am certainly not saying that there is no place for ultrasound in the field of breast-cancer detection. Ultrasound will be able to demonstrate many cases of breast cancer and is an excellent technique for determining whether a breast mass is cystic (contains fluid) or solid. At present, ultrasound should be thought of as a useful supplement to, rather than replacement for, mammography.

THERMOGRAPHY

Thermography is based on the principle that the blood flow to tumors is different from the blood flow to normal tissue, resulting in an alteration in temperature patterns at an area harboring a tumor. Therefore, an area with a malignancy will frequently produce an abnormal thermographic pattern.

Unfortunately, the technique of thermography in its present state is quite inaccurate and cannot currently be considered an adequate screening technique by itself. Thermograms are very imprecise, and have a high false-negative rate (a normal thermogram when a tumor is actually present) and a high false-positive rate (an abnormal thermogram, suggestive of a tumor, when none is present).

Thermography is most likely to detect large tumors, which can be palpated (felt) by the patient or physician, and is least likely to detect the very early cancers. It has been estimated that as many as forty to fifty percent of small tumors that can be detected by mammography may be missed in thermography. If thermography is used in conjunction with mammography, it may possibly assist in the diagnosis of a breast cancer undetected by either mammography or physical examination, but this is not very likely.

The technique of thermography involves no known risks in itself. However, a tumor missed by thermography and thus not diagnosed may prove fatal, or will at least have reached a more advanced stage by the time it is detected. And a woman with a false-positive thermogram may undergo considerable psychological stress, besides incurring the discomfort and expense of several other medical procedures to rule out a tumor.

There is, of course, hope that the technique of thermography will be refined in the future, but at present it is *not* an adequate substitute for mammography; even if your doctor recommends thermography, you probably should also have mammography performed, at the intervals outlined earlier in this chapter.

DIAPHANOGRAPHY

Diaphanography (breast transillumination) is a technique in which light, a large portion of which is near infrared wavelengths, is passed through the breast tissue. Breast cancer, if present, will appear as a dark mass. Diaphanography is more likely to miss small breast cancers. This technique still requires more research to demonstrate precisely its clinical applications and accuracy.

COMPUTERIZED AXIAL TOMOGRAPHY (CT)

Although the availability of CT scanning has had a major impact in many fields of medical practice, such as aiding in the diagnosis of brain abnormalities and masses in the abdomen, it does not appear to be significantly useful for breast-cancer screening. The radiation exposure it entails is too great for this technique to be employed for routine screening.

NUCLEAR MAGNETIC RESONANCE IMAGING (NMR)

Nuclear magnetic resonance imaging is a very promising new technique, though many of its clinical applications are still somewhat experimental. It is noninvasive (nothing is placed inside the body), and does not produce radiation exposure. However, since it is so new, it is possible that it results in other toxicities and side effects that have not yet been discovered.

With NMR, the tissue is exposed to an external magnetic field, with oscillating radiowaves. This causes hydrogen nuclei in the body to resonate. The energy that is radiated back by the resonating hydrogen nuclei will then be displayed as the NMR image. The NMR picture will indicate which areas have the greatest hydrogen ion densities, and will be able to indicate areas that are potentially abnormal.

It is at present impossible to be certain whether NMR will be useful for breast cancer screening programs, but it may hold promise.

In summary, breast cancer screening programs have saved thousands of lives and will continue to save hundreds of thousands more. On rare occasion, breast cancers develop so rapidly that even the woman who has been involved in a screening program will not be diagnosed until she has an advanced disease, but this is quite unusual. Ideally, the aim of breast cancer screening is to diagnose tumors while they are in their earliest state and have the greatest likelihood of being curable. In addition, a large body of evidence is accumulating that indicates that if a breast cancer is diagnosed early enough, it can probably be cured by merely removing the breast cancer and the tissue immediately surrounding it plus lymph nodes in the axilla (underarm) and radiating the breast, without removing the breast itself. The cosmetic results with this procedure are excellent; in many cases the breast that had previously harbored a cancer has a completely normal appearance. This is not true when breast cancer is diagnosed in an advanced state.

To reiterate one set of guidelines for the early detection of breast cancer:

1. From the age of twenty on, perform monthly breast self-examination.

2. Breast examination by a doctor should be done at least annually once a woman reaches the age of thirty-five, and should probably be done even more often if the woman is at very high risk of developing breast cancer. Examination by a physician should begin when a woman is twenty and should be performed at least once every three years between the ages of twenty and thirty-five. I believe that a woman who is at high risk of developing breast cancer, or is being seen by a doctor for any other reasons, should have at least annual breast examinations by a physician, from the age of twenty onward. Your personal physician, however, is best able to advise you on how often to be examined, given your unique medical and family history.

3. A baseline mammography should be performed at some time between the ages of thirty-five and forty, depending upon a woman's risk factors. These risk factors will guide her doctor in deciding how frequently mammography should be performed when she is between the ages of forty and forty-nine. Annual mammography is recommended for women from the age of fifty onward.

4. Any abnormality that a woman finds in her breast should be reported immediately to her physician.

I urge you to participate in breast cancer screening. Read the chapter on breast self-examination and perform it monthly. Have your breasts examined by your doctor, and discuss mammography with him or her, so that you understand the procedure and its potential risks and benefits. Once you understand it thoroughly, I think you will want to participate fully in a complete screening program.

CHAPTER IV

Breast Self-Examination

Once a woman reaches the age of twenty, she should examine her breasts monthly. The examination takes only a few minutes and costs nothing. Not examining your breasts, on the other hand, may cost you your life.

Breast self-examination should be done at a routine time each month. For women who are having menstrual periods, the examination should be done approximately seven days after the onset of your period. At this time of the month (the proliferative phase of the menstrual cycle), the breasts are usually not swollen or tender; later in the menstrual cycle the breasts are more likely to feel somewhat irregular, and normal monthly variations in the breasts are more likely to be misinterpreted as suspicious masses. If you are no longer menstruating, examine your breasts on the first day of each month.

Breast self-examination consists of three steps, each of which is quite important, and none of which should ever be omitted. Once you have made the proper commitment to examine your breasts every month, you should try to do it as meticulously as possible, so that even the earliest perceivable abnormality will not escape your detection.

Step one is to examine your breasts while you are showering (or in the tub, if you do not take showers). Use your right hand to examine your left breast and your left hand to examine your right breast. Using the flat part of your fingers, touch every portion of your breast tissue. You are searching for nodules, lumps, or anything that feels irregular. Examine each armpit as well. Push high into the armpit with the fingers of the opposite hand, searching for lymph nodes.

Step two is to examine your breasts visually without touching them. Sit in front of a mirror. Begin by looking at your breasts while your arms are at your sides. You are looking for anything in your breasts that was not present on previous examinations—changes in skin color, changes in contour, dimpling, nipple retraction, breast swelling, or an unusual asymmetry (most women's breasts do not match identically, but an alteration in the asymmetry may be significant). Once you have looked at your breasts with your arms at your sides, raise your arms straight above your head, and again look for the abnormal findings previously described. Finally, put your hands on your hips and push them tightly into your hips, so that your chest muscles are flexed. You are again looking for the aforementioned abnormalities. Then, examine your breasts as you did in the shower.

The third and final step is an examination while you are lying down on your back. To examine your left breast, place a pillow under your left shoulder. Then, with the flat part of the fingers of your right hand, feel every portion of your breast tissue in a systematic fashion.

One good way to examine the entire breast properly is to start at the outermost top of the breast and move your hand in a circular fashion around the 360 degrees of the entire outer breast. Then move in one inch toward the nipple, and again feel 360 degrees around the entire circle of breast tissue. Then move in another inch and do the same. Continue moving in, an inch at a time, until all the breast tissue, including the nipple, has been examined. In other words, if your breast is five inches in diameter, you should examine your breast tissue by making circles that are five inches in diameter, four inches in diameter, three inches, two inches, and one inch, and then examining the tissue under the nipple.

Repeat the procedure for your right breast, using a pillow under your right shoulder, and your left hand to examine the right breast.

Next, squeeze your nipple to look for discharge. If any nipple discharge is present, it may represent an abnormality. Finally, with your right arm relaxed and limp, place your left hand deep into your right armpit (and vice versa). You are feeling for any indication of swelling or nodules.

The first few times a woman performs breast self-examination it almost always seems cumbersome and confusing. Please do not be discouraged if the exam seems awkward, or if you are positive you feel an abnormality and your doctor says it is just normal breast tissue. This sense of unfamiliarity with the technique is very common at first, but after a few months it will be second nature to you. After two or three examinations, you will have an excellent sense of what your breasts feel like and what is normal for you. In fact, since you are examining your breasts every month, and your doctor is probably only examining them once a year, it is likely that you would notice an abnormality even before your doctor would.

When you are first learning how to examine your breasts, it may be helpful to go through the physical steps while your doctor (or the nurse or medical assistant) is watching.

That way you can feel reassured that you are performing the examination properly, and your physician can make certain that you are indeed performing it correctly.

Of course, anything you discover while performing breast self-examination that is not clearly normal must be evaluated immediately by your physician. Don't be alarmed: often these findings are just benign changes in the breast. Remember not to be embarrassed if the doctor tells you that what you have felt is just within the limits of normal, and don't be shy in the future about reporting to your physician anything you notice that is not clearly normal. Only the doctor has the expertise to determine whether what you have found is a potential indicator of malignancy.

Breast self-examination is easy to learn, is quick and simple to perform, and costs nothing. Of course, omitting the examination is also quite simple (as evidenced by the fact that, despite all the media attention it has received, most American women still do not examine their breasts). However, there is a great potential cost related to the omission of breast self-examination—it may cost hundreds of thousands of lives.

CHAPTER V

If a Lump Is Found

You have done your job diligently and been involved in a careful screening program. Each month you have methodically examined your breasts, meticulously looking for a lump while simultaneously praying that you would not find one. Each month you have been relieved to find your fears unwarranted.

Unfortunately, one month the examination feels a little different. You suspect that there is a lump. Do not become paralyzed with anxiety. The reason for examining your breasts so painstakingly is to locate any potential problems as early as possible. With breast masses, trouble does not come because you were looking for it. If a problem exists, it will be there whether or not you search for it, but searching for it, identifying the problem if it is present, and acting upon it as soon as possible will afford you the greatest opportunity to lose neither your breast nor your life.

If you examine your breast and find a lump, make an appointment to see your doctor within the next several days. To do anything else would negate the value of your entire self-examination program. Until you visit your physician, your anxiety level is likely to be extremely high. Do not deal with this anxiety by denying that there may be a problem and procrastinating. The anxiety is meant to work for you, pushing you to seek medical advice as soon as possible.

There is a good chance that what you have found is absolutely benign. If so, having your doctor confirm this will immediately alleviate your anxiety. On the other hand, if you have found a very early malignancy, seeking attention right away will give you the greatest opportunity to have the best outcome: to be cured and also to keep your breast.

Although every situation is somewhat different, based on your individual physical examination and medical data, the following is a general outline of what might happen when a woman consults a physician because she has palpated a breast mass. The discussion that follows is of course just one possible scenario. Remember that what many women believe to be new findings turn out to be merely part of the normal breast tissue and require no biopsy at all. Again, if your doctor determines that what you have found is a normal variant not requiring a biopsy, you must never feel distressed at being overly cautious. It is your job to be meticulous in your self-examination; that is the purpose of the program. Continue as vigorously and enthusiastically as ever with your monthly breast self-examination.

Let us return now to the woman who has palpated a lump and is seeking medical advice. If the woman is unknown to the doctor, a complete, detailed medical history will be taken and a careful physical examination will be performed. This will probably include a general examination in addition to a very thorough breast examination.

Frequently, the physician will want a mammography done, both to evaluate the area in question and also to study all other areas of both breasts. It is important to realize that a negative mammography does not guarantee the absence of a malignancy. Although mammography is an excellent tool, it is not one-hundred-percent accurate. Therefore, if a physician feels a breast mass, a biopsy or an aspiration may be warranted even if a mammography has been performed and is interpreted as being normal.

Although most physicians do not advise ultrasound for screening purposes, it is often useful once a mass has been found, since the technique is excellent at differentiating cystic from solid lesions.

If the breast mass is cystic, and the mammography is not suggestive of a malignancy, the doctor will probably perform what is called a "needle aspiration." This procedure is done in the office and for most women produces only slight discomfort. A needle is placed into the cyst and all the fluid is withdrawn, so that the cyst completely collapses. The physician may send the fluid to a cytologist, who looks under the microscope to attempt to identify any malignant cells.

Once a cyst has been aspirated, a woman must return to her doctor for a series of evaluations to make sure it does not recur; if the cyst does reappear, this may signify that there is a more serious problem. In many cases, the breast mass a woman finds is merely a benign cyst. The fluid is removed, the cyst fully collapses, there are no malignant cells in the fluid, and upon repeated examination by the physician the cyst does not recur.

There are circumstances under which even an apparent cyst must be biopsied, however. If the fluid is bloody, a biopsy is usually warranted. If malignant cells are found in the fluid that has been removed, a biopsy must certainly be done. If the mass does not fully disappear once the fluid has been removed, or if the mass recurs under careful observation, a biopsy must also be performed.

There are several additional reasons why a doctor might suggest a breast biopsy. These include the presence of a solid breast mass, a bloody nipple discharge, or a persistently encrusted or ulcerated nipple. Even in the absence of a palpable breast mass, if a mammography turns up an area suspicious of being malignant, the physician will need to perform a breast biopsy. It is important not to ignore such a finding on mammography, since under these circumstances a breast cancer might be diagnosed so early that it would be nonpalpable, therefore having an excellent prognosis and, once again, much improving the woman's chance to be cured without losing her breast. If a physician finds an enlarged lymph node in the underarm, a biopsy might be suggested even if the mammography is normal and no breast mass is palpated.

Most women who have been scheduled for a breast biopsy are enormously anxious about the procedure. Usually, the anxiety is not related to the operation itself but, rather, to their fear about the outcome: they are afraid the lesion will be discovered to be malignant. Quite often a breast biopsy is performed and the tissue is found benign, an outcome that obviously produces an enormous sense of elation and relief. Some women do not resume a program of breast cancer screening following a biopsy. The experience has provoked so much anxiety for them that they attempt to blot it from memory by avoiding the issue. This is clearly a mistake. Women who have had certain types of benign breast masses may be at increased risk of subsequently developing a breast cancer.

If you need a breast biopsy, although the procedure is sometimes performed in the doctor's office, your doctor may recommend that it be done in the hospital. During the past few years it has become common, particularly for young, healthy women who appear to have benign tumors, to have the breast biopsy performed as "ambulatory surgery." This means that you will only be at the hospital, or ambulatory surgery center, for several hours and will not have to stay overnight. On the other hand, your physician might have a reason for recommending that your biopsy be performed while you are an in-patient, particularly if you have other serious medical problems or if there is a significant likelihood that the tumor is malignant.

Many years ago it was considered essentially standard procedure for a woman about to undergo a breast biopsy to test for a malignant lesion to sign a consent for both the breast biopsy and a possible mastectomy. Women would routinely be anesthetized for a breast biopsy not knowing whether they were going to wake up with or without the breast. This could add extensive psychological trauma to an already exceedingly traumatic situation. If your doctor asks you to sign a consent for a breast biopsy plus a possible mastectomy, make sure that you have fully considered the options first. Giving such a consent is not automatic, and you definitely have the right to question the doctor and to make sure this is truly what you wish done.

In 1978, Nancy Winters, a thirty-seven-year-old divorced schoolteacher, found a mass the size of a large pea in the upper outer portion of her right breast. Nancy scheduled an appointment with her gynecologist a few days later. The gynecologist, concerned about the possibility of a malignancy, sent Nancy for a mammography the next day. She also gave her the names of three breast surgeons in the city. The day after the mammography was done, Nancy saw a surgeon. He told her that both the mass and the mammography were suspicious, and that surgery would be necessary.

One week later, Nancy was in the hospital. She was seen first by a nurse and then by the resident physician. After the resident had obtained a complete medical history and performed a physical examination, he asked Nancy to sign a consent for surgery. She was very upset when she realized that she was being asked to sign her consent not only for a biopsy of the right breast, but for a possible right modified radical mastectomy as well. The resident told Nancy that this was standard procedure, and he seemed quite annoyed when she refused to sign the form. Nancy said that she was absolutely unwilling to sign the consent for mastectomy, and that she would discuss this further with her surgeon when he came to see her that evening.

When the doctor spoke with Nancy, she told him that she was willing only to have a biopsy to find out if the mass was malignant. The doctor explained to her that if the mass was found to be malignant, he would be recommending that she have a mastectomy, so it seemed pointless for her to have two anesthetics, one for the biopsy and the other for the mastectomy. Since Nancy was not convinced that signing consent for a mastectomy was the right thing to do, she agreed only to the biopsy, which was done the following day.

Unfortunately, as the doctor had expected, the breast mass was malignant. The doctor advised Nancy to have a modified radical mastectomy. In her city and, in fact, in most of the country, this was considered to be the best way to cure her tumor. Within a few days, Nancy had spoken with several friends and done a lot of reading. She found that close by, in Boston, doctors were offering women with small breast cancers the option of having just the lump and the lymph nodes removed. They were treating the malignancy with radiation and not removing the breast. Nancy contacted the doctors in Boston. They explained to her that although there was not yet enough experience to be certain, they believed that radiation could be equally as effective as surgery in curing her malignancy. They explained to her that there was much that was not yet known, and discussed with her all the possible risks and benefits of both radiation and surgery.

Nancy considered the two therapies carefully and opted for radiation. After the tumor was excised and lymph nodes were removed, radiation was administered to her breast. Eight years later, she's still happy that she made a decision she feels was right for her.

There exist certain circumstances under which it is appropriate for a breast biopsy and a mastectomy to be done under one anesthetic. For instance, an elderly woman with a large breast mass and many enlarged lymph nodes might be a good candidate, especially if she is unwilling to have the biopsy with only local anesthesia. Assuming she agrees that if the tumor is malignant she will have a mastectomy, it would be wiser to anesthetize her only once than to re-anesthetize her for a mastectomy. In general, however, performing a breast biopsy and a mastectomy under one anesthetic is no longer considered standard procedure.

What is somewhat more likely to happen now is that a woman who has a breast mass will have a breast biopsy done without signing a consent for a mastectomy. If the lesion if benign, she will not have had to undergo that trauma. After surgery, she will resume her breast cancer screening program. If a diagnosis of malignancy is made, her doctor will present the therapeutic options to her and discuss them with her. It is now the law in several states that a woman who has breast cancer must have the various types of acceptable therapy presented to her before she has her treatment.

I think it is important for women to understand fully what options are available to them, and I believe that most doctors are pleased to discuss all the appropriate choices (when there are acceptable choices to be made) and data with the patient. Unfortunately, there are still gaps in what is known, because the data are not yet available, and this can cloud the issues. For instance, it is established that, if a woman has a small breast cancer (less than four centimeters in diameter) and there is no tumor in the lymph nodes, she is equally likely to be alive and healthy several years later whether she is treated with a modified radical mastectomy or with removal of the lump, removal of lymph nodes, and radiation therapy. However, what has not yet been demonstrated to the satisfaction of all is whether she is equally likely to be alive and healthy twenty years later. Since it is known that breast cancers can recur a long time after the original occurrence, this is quite an important issue to clarify. We don't yet know whether the absolute chance of cure will be the same over the long range, regardless of which treatment is chosen. Many doctors, myself included, do believe that for early breast cancer, removal of the lump and lymph nodes followed by radiation therapy will result in the same probability of cure as will modified radical mastectomy. However, this is not yet an absolutely proven scientific fact.

I frequently lecture to groups of physicians, and one of the areas obviously of greatest concern to me, and therefore one I often discuss, is the management of breast cancer without resorting to mastectomy. As I have just mentioned, all the data are not yet available as to whether the long-range prognosis will be identical regardless of whether the woman is treated with mastectomy or with lump removal and radiation therapy. However, most of the data we do have suggest that for women who have early breast cancer, the survival rate will be the same with either therapy. I firmly believe, therefore, that the doctor should provide the patient who has breast cancer with all the available information on her therapeutic options, and that the woman should decide, based upon this information, which of them is reasonable, given her personal situation.

When I presented this point of view during one lecture, I was interrupted by a physician who said, "How can we let the patient decide when we ourselves have no idea as to which choice is better?" I think this is precisely the point. When there *is* clearly only one appropriate therapeutic option available to a patient, then I as a physician must make that known to her and advise her that this is the only correct medical decision to be made. On the other hand, if two reasonable therapeutic options are available, these should be presented to the patient along with information on the risks and benefits of each choice. When there is a reasonable medical choice to be made, it is fully appropriate that the patient make that choice. Fortunately, in 1987, this conviction is held by the vast majority of doctors.

As patients, you should be working with your physicians. The physician should be providing information, guidance, and advice. When the decision is clear-cut, the physician should tell you so. Depending on the size of the tumor, its location, its involvement of the chest wall, skin, or lymph nodes, or the presence of distant metastases, there may be only one appropriate therapeutic regimen. It is not reasonable to expect that a doctor can be persuaded to carry out a treatment course that is inferior or untested, or in which he or she does not believe. However, you as the patient obviously have the right to know why, in your particular situation, your doctor feels there is only one acceptable plan of therapy.

Phyllis Johnson is a thin, married thirty-four-year-old administrative assistant who noticed a grape-sized mass in her breast while she was shopping for lingerie. A few relatives of hers had had breast cancer, but they had been much older when it occurred, so she felt that this could not possibly be her problem, and she put it out of her mind.

Several months later, her husband mentioned to her that he felt a hardness in her breast and asked her whether she had been to the doctor. She told him she was sure it was nothing. However, later that evening, when she was alone, she fearfully touched the area and realized that the mass was quite a bit larger than when she had first noticed it. Though she became very anxious, she decided that it must be a large premenstrual cyst, and that she would watch it during the next month or so.

Phyllis was under enormous stress at work, faced with several end-of-year reports to prepare. She put the breast problem out of her thoughts.

It wasn't until several more months had passed that Phyllis became so frightened she finally decided to take some action. Getting out of the shower, she caught a glimpse of her breast in the full-length mirror. It appeared distorted. When she felt her breast, there was a mass almost the size of a tennis ball.

Panic-stricken, she went to see her doctor. The mass turned out to be a very large cancer. In addition, the tumor had spread to several lymph nodes in her underarm.

The doctor told Phyllis that she would require a mastectomy and then chemotherapy. Phyllis told her doctor that she had read about a new operation in which breast cancer could be cured by removing the tumor mass plus lymph nodes in the underarm, but preserving the breast and treating the tumor with radiation. Although the doctor had performed that operation many times, and was a strong supporter of the concept of curing breast cancer while keeping the breast intact, he told Phyllis that this was not a reasonable approach to her particular situation. He explained to her that because her tumor was so large, radiation was unlikely to be able to eradicate it. Besides, the tumor had replaced such a large proportion of her breast that the cosmetic result of a lumpectomy (removal of the tumor alone) would be poor anyway, because there would be almost no remaining breast tissue once the tumor mass was removed. He said that he could not do a lumpectomy, because he felt that it was the wrong operation.

When Phyllis remained adamant about wanting a lumpectomy, the doctor suggested that she seek other opinions, both from radiation therapists and from surgeons. Phyllis proceeded to do this. However, all the physicians with whom she had consultations independently gave her the same advice as her own doctor.

Under some circumstances, there really is no good therapeutic option other than mastectomy. However, when there are choices to be made, you and your doctor should work together to decide what is right for you. Your physician will provide you with all the information regarding the possible treatment plans and their risks and benefits. If the doctor feels that one treatment plan is preferable, he or she will let you know which it is and why it is preferred. But, I repeat, when there is a choice to be made, it is ultimately you, the patient, who must make it.

A woman who has been told she has a malignancy is obviously in an extremely vulnerable position. She must deal with an enormous range of emotions and an inordinate amount of pressure. In such a situation, any person, man or woman, may find it difficult to think clearly and evaluate the options with logic. Once a physician tells a woman that she has a malignancy, even if the doctor assumed it is his or her solemn responsibility to help a woman understand totally the risks and benefits of all available alternatives, it may be difficult to transmit this information at the time and have the patient absorb it fully. It is obvious that the data regarding the optimal therapy for early breast cancer are controversial, complicated, and detailed. It is equally apparent that people frequently find it difficult to comprehend fully such complex information, especially if it was previously totally foreign to them, and when they are under such unusual stress.

If you are reading this book now, and if at some point your doctor must describe to you treatment alternatives for breast cancer, the information will not be foreign to you. You will have considerable depth and breadth in your understanding of the disease and its treatment. One of my reasons for writing this book, and one of the many reasons for your reading it, is that, should you or one of your friends develop a breast cancer, you will not become paralyzed at this point (as so many millions of women have been).

Once the diagnosis of breast cancer is made, the doctor will probably continue to discuss options for therapy. Before you start asking questions, listen carefully to all that the doctor has to say.

Then do start asking questions. Lots of questions. Ask about all the therapeutic options as they apply to your particular tumor, because there are great variations in what to expect, depending upon its size, location, involvement of the skin, involvement of the chest wall, presence of tumor in lymph nodes, appearance of the tumor under the microscope, etc., etc., etc. You don't want to know about any other woman's tumor; you want to know about yours.

So ask very carefully what, for your particular situation, are all the acceptable therapies, and what are the potential risks and benefits of each. What is the likelihood of your being cured? What are the probable cosmetic results? What are the potential side effects?

Listen carefully. There is no formula answer, and the solution may be different for each woman. For example, even if data eventually become available which convince all physicians that the chance of a long-term cure for the woman who has a very small breast cancer is the same whether the woman undergoes a modified radical mastectomy or the removal of only the lump and lymph nodes and subsequent radiation, modified radical mastectomy might still be appropriate therapy for certain women with small breast tumors. If a woman has exceedingly small breasts, her cosmetic result might actually be better with modified radical mastectomy and breast reconstruction than with lumpectomy, since lumpectomy might cause considerable distortion to a very small breast. On the other hand, some radiation therapists feel that the best results with lumpectomy and radiation are for women whose breasts are not exceedingly large. They find that when the breasts are very large, the radiation may cause retraction and fibrosis (deposits of fibrous tissue), resulting in some asymmetry and changes in consistency.

The point I am making is that you must understand not just what is appropriate for women in general, but, more important, what is best for you. Ask specific questions, listen carefully to the answers, and then ask more questions. Continue asking questions until you are satisfied that you understand all you need and want to know about your problem.

It is often helpful to have another person sit in on this meeting with your doctor. I don't believe that this person should be there to make the decision for you: I think it must be your decision, because it is your body and your life. However, with the degree of anxiety that is almost always present in such a situation, you may well find it helpful to have someone else present with whom you can review all the information later on. This discussion with your physician is of such importance, and often so emotional, that it may be difficult in the ensuing days to remember some of the very complex, detailed points.

This conversation with your physician should be mutually supportive. You will be working together to try to determine the course that is most likely to give you the best outcome with regard to cancer cure, psychological response, physical function, and aesthetics. You must listen to all the data that the doctor has (remembering that a great deal is still not known), and then weigh which variables are most important to you. Only you really know what trade-offs you are willing to make.

At present, modified radical mastectomy is still considered by some to be the standard, tried-and-true therapy. Whereas lumpectomy, lymph-node removal, and radiation seem to offer the same opportunity for cure for many groups of women, some doctors think this is not fully proved. Only you can decide whether going along with more traditional therapy is right for you, or whether you are willing to take what may be construed by some as somewhat more of a risk (though it may not be) to preserve your breast. Ultimately, the woman must make her own decision.

For the woman who does decide on mastectomy, I believe that the options for breast reconstruction should be discussed before surgery. Knowing that the breast can be reconstructed, and how attractively it can be done, can offer very powerful emotional and psychological support.

To summarize, once a lump has been found in a woman's breast, the first step is to determine its cause. This will usually entail a mammography, possibly a breast ultrasound, and then probably the aspiration and/or biopsy of the mass.

If the lesion is benign, it is still important that you continue to see your doctor for follow-up exactly as he or she has advised, and that you continue your screening program.

If breast cancer is found, you will need several blood studies and a chest X-ray. Depending on your doctor's clinical evaluation of the extent of the breast cancer and the results of the blood studies, he or she may feel that a few other radiologic tests are required, most commonly a bone scan, and perhaps a liver scan. These painless tests will help the physician ascertain that the cancer has spread neither to the bones nor to the liver, two potential areas of breast cancer metastases.

Once your doctor has evaluated the size and characteristics of the tumor and determined, to the extent possible, whether metastases have occurred, he or she will be able to discuss therapeutic options with you. Listen very carefully, ask questions, and make certain that you understand all the risks, benefits, and alternatives. No patient should ever be uncomfortable about asking any question, or even asking the same question more than once.

Work together with your physician to arrive at your decision. You should feel that you and your doctor are working together as a team with a single goal, for you to get well. However, since it is your body and your life, only you have the privilege of ultimately making the decision.

Between now and your surgery, and in the months that follow, you will experience a wide range of emotions. All of the negative emotions will surface. Having breast cancer can't help being an enormous strain, and for most women it is better for them to accept their feelings and work them through, rather than to try to deny that they exist.

However, once you have experienced the negative and have accepted what has happened, you should also feel hope. Try to resume your life in a positive way. Remember that most women who have breast cancer are cured. Hope and believe that you will be one of them.

Except for continuing to go for your physical and X-ray examinations exactly as your doctor has instructed, try not to keep your former tumor in the forefront of your thoughts. That was the past. You endured the physical and emotional strain of the past because the future was important to you. There is a good likelihood that you will be cured, but the cure is all the more valuable if you are enjoying the life it has allowed you.

Almost all the women I have treated for gynecologic malignancy have approached their disease with great courage. They have accepted the diagnosis, undergone the discomforts of treatment, and worked with me to help them be cured. Although I have always worked very hard with my patients, they are the ones who have had the endurance, bravery, and will to accept the therapy and the challenge of overcoming the illness.

After the initial treatment for a malignancy, I tell each patient what her regimen for follow-up visits should be, what types of problems she must be on the alert for, and under what circumstances she must notify me.

Some women follow my instructions and then resume all the day-to-day pleasures of living. They reintegrate themselves with their families, friends, and jobs. While it's probably impossible for them to forget that they have had cancer, they consider it essentially a problem in the past tense. I'm certain that they occasionally worry about the possibility of recurrence, but they consider themselves whole and cured and live in the present. Some women even appreciate life's pleasures more following their confrontation with such a serious medical problem.

I worry so much about the woman at the other extreme, the woman who has fought with equal courage to overcome her disease, but who lives with constant fear that each new day brings with it the possibility of recurrent tumor. This woman has endured so much in order to live, but never really resumes the pleasures that she has bravely fought to retain. It is painful for me as a doctor and a friend to watch someone who is probably physically cured of her disease continue to carry such emotional weight each minute of her life.

Obviously, some women will develop recurrent disease and will ultimately have the very arduous task of dealing with the physical and emotional traumas this brings. However, many, many women will be cured by their initial therapy.

I believe that the best thing a woman who has completed treatment for a malignancy can do is to accept that she has had cancer and must continue to have checkups. However, she should, as much as possible, consider the disease in the past tense and not let it interfere with the joys and the other challenges that a full, active life will bring.

CHAPTER VI

Conservative Therapy for Breast Cancer (Can You Save Your Breast and Still Save Your Life?)

When a woman is diagnosed as having breast cancer, there are two major issues confronting her. One is that she has just been told she has a malignancy—a devastating fact for any man or woman to assimilate. But the other is that she must face the possibility of a major surgical procedure that may affect her body image and her self-image as a sexual being. Most women who have had a mastectomy are eventually able to cope with the diagnosis and with the operation, and to accept the situation, but almost all confronted with it feel some threat to their sense of their own sexuality. Unfortunately, some are never able fully to recover their former self-image, let alone their sense of sexual desirability.

If a woman with breast cancer could be cured without having a mastectomy, she would at least have one less trauma to cope with. If she could preserve her silhouette and be cured without incurring significant physical change, she would almost certainly experience less psychological stress.

The question therefore is: can we offer a woman with breast cancer the same opportunity for cure if we remove the tumor lump and a small amount of surrounding breast tissue (a surgical procedure known as tylectomy or lumpectomy), remove lymph nodes in her underarm, and radiate the breast as we can with some form of mastectomy? A second important question is: will the cosmetic results with lumpectomy and radiation be a significant improvement over those with mastectomy?

At present, some physicians feel that there are not enough thoroughly evaluated prospective scientific data to establish definitively whether we can produce the same cure rates with lumpectomy and radiation as can be produced with mastectomy. However, there are data available that strongly suggest that we can, particularly for women who have only small tumors. Dr. Umberto Veronesi, an Italian physician from the National Tumor Institute in Milan, who has been a pioneer in new methods of breast cancer treatment, has found that for women with small tumors (those less than two centimeters in size that clinically do not appear to have tumor involving lymph nodes), removing the quadrant of the breast that harbors the malignancy, plus removing the lymph nodes in the underarm on the affected side, and then treating the involved area with radiation has so far resulted in equivalent survival rates to those achieved by women who have been treated by radical mastectomy (an operation in which the breast is removed). This study, which Dr. Veronesi and his associates conducted between 1973 and 1980, was reported in the prestigious *New England Journal of Medicine* in July 1981.

There are three significant points that one must be careful to consider in looking at these results. The first is that when these data were evaluated, the women had been followed for less than ten years after therapy. This is not a long enough period on which to base definitive conclusions regarding breast cancer cures, since breast cancer is a disease in which one may see late recurrences—not infrequently, more than a dozen years following therapy.

The second significant consideration is the importance of removing lymph nodes from the underarm. If a patient is to be treated without mastectomy, most physicians feel that these lymph nodes should still be removed, since if the tumor has spread to the lymph nodes, the woman should have further therapy so that she can still have a fair opportunity to be cured.

The final, extremely important point about Veronesi's data is that they concern women who have small tumors. This again underscores the major importance of diagnosing a tumor when it is small, and stresses the significance of screening by breast self-examination, physician examination, and mammography. The patient who is diligent in her breast cancer screening regimen and has a breast cancer found when it is quite small may be able to be cured of the malignancy without sacrificing her breast. On the other hand, the woman who, through fear or ignorance, dismisses the problem until a large breast mass is apparent will not only be less likely to be cured, but is less likely to be a candidate for breast conservation as well. Although there are instances in which women who are regularly screened for breast cancer develop large, aggressive tumors, these are the exception.

Another study that supports conservation of the breast for patients whose breast cancer is diagnosed early was reported by Dr. Bernard Fisher in the *New England Journal of Medicine* in 1985. His initial data indicated that the early survival rates (survival during the first several years) would be the same for women with breast cancers up to four centimeters in size whether they were treated by mastectomy or by removal of the cancer and dissection of lymph nodes with subsequent radiation therapy, thus preserving the breast. In his study, all patients who had tumor in lymph nodes, whether or not they had a mastectomy, received chemotherapy.

This study is exciting and the information encouraging. However, Dr. Fisher's patients had been followed, on average, for less than four years from the time of therapy. Again, since breast cancer may recur a dozen years or more after the initial tumor has been treated, he is unable to say whether the ultimate likelihood of being cured will be the same for his patients whether they have been treated by mastectomy or with preservation of the breast and radiation therapy. Still, his initial findings are encouraging and his long-term data are eagerly awaited.

Although some women who have larger breast cancers have been treated without resorting to mastectomy, the problems arising here are greater. The larger the malignancy, the greater the amount of the breast that will have to be removed even in a lumpectomy operation, and the smaller the chance of an acceptable cosmetic result. In addition, the larger the malignancy, the greater the likelihood that by the time of diagnosis the disease will already have metastasized (spread) to the lymph nodes and perhaps elsewhere. A patient to whom this has happened will require further therapy, usually chemotherapy, and will have to tolerate its side effects—in addition to having a significantly diminished chance for cure.

Even if the cure rates for the treatment of breast cancer by lumpectomy, lymph node removal, and radiation can be definitively proved to be the same as the cure rates with mastectomy, which I believe will probably be the case, there are still some potential problems that must be faced in considering lumpectomy and lymph node removal plus radiation therapy.

Since the option of conservative surgery plus radiation is usually chosen in an attempt to achieve a good cosmetic effect, one significant problem is that this cannot always be achieved. I have examined some women who have had lumpectomy, lymph node removal, and radiation in whom the cosmetic results are so excellent that, even knowing that the patient has been treated for a breast cancer, I could not see any significant difference between her two breasts. And for most women treated with lumpectomy and radiation, the cosmetic results are quite good. However, for a woman who has either exceedingly small breasts, very large breasts, or a large tumor, the cosmetic result may be poor. While not all women are completely satisfied with the cosmetic results, most are quite pleased.

There are other potential problems to be considered when radiating the breast, although there is a very small chance of their ensuing. Theoretically, radiation therapy to the breast may itself be carcinogenic and could cause a second breast cancer. Several authorities feel that this is extremely unlikely, since women who have been treated with radiation for breast cancer have not yet been shown to have an increased incidence of cancer in the other breast, when compared with women who have been treated surgically.

Other potential problems that occur infrequently when treating the breast with radiation include the possible development of scarring of the lung and a possible subsequent diminution of the blood flow through the coronary arteries, which supply the heart with blood, potentially producing heart disease.

The radiation may also cause a lowering of the white-blood-cell count and platelet count, since these cells are produced in the bone marrow, which will be receiving some radiation in the course of treatment. White blood cells are needed to ward off infection; platelets play an important role in helping the blood to clot. If the white blood-cell count or platelet count is lowered, it may be more difficult subsequently to give chemotherapy if required, since chemotherapy will further diminish the number of white blood cells and platelets.

Upon occasion, a woman who has been treated by lumpectomy and radiation therapy will develop a recurrent tumor in the radiated breast. If the recurrent disease is localized to the breast, the patient can often be cured by mastectomy. The larger the tumor is when first diagnosed, the greater the probability of a local recurrence in the breast following lumpectomy and radiation, and of the eventual need for a mastectomy. Again we see that the woman who is most likely to benefit from conservative therapy and achieve a good cosmetic result is the woman who is properly screened, who performs breast self-examination, and who seeks medical attention immediately for any abnormal findings, since this is the woman in whom a breast cancer is most likely to be diagnosed while it is still small.

In summary, the answer to the question of whether a woman with breast cancer can save her breast and save her life is yes. Whether treatment without mastectomy will produce the same cure rates as removal of the breast has not yet been answered with one-hundred-percent certainty, but there is a significant body of data available to indicate that the answer to that question will also probably be yes. Women who have been followed for ten years after therapy for breast cancer seem to have the same survival statistics whether they have been treated by removal of the lump and lymph nodes followed by radiation or by modified radical mastectomy. As has been mentioned, since breast cancer may recur at intervals of greater than ten years following initial therapy, it would be even more reassuring if the patients had been followed for longer periods of time.

At present in the United States, what is still regarded by some doctors to be the traditional, standard therapy for breast cancer is modified radical mastectomy. However, just because it has been considered the standard therapy does not really prove that it is better than alternative therapies. Conservative therapy by lumpectomy, lymph node removal, and radiation may not merely produce the identical cure rate but may do so with less cosmetic and psychological trauma.

How does a woman with breast cancer decide what therapy is appropriate for her? Although this should only be done on the basis of correct and complete information, it unfortunately is usually done in a period of great stress, with haste, and before complete information has been collected or assimilated. Your best assets are a well-educated, well-informed, caring physician who takes the time to provide proper counseling and a thorough discussion of the risks, benefits, and alternatives as they apply to your particular situation, and your own capability to evaluate logically the information that you have obtained, both from your doctor and through your reading. Probably no one knows you as well as you know yourself. This means you are the one who is best able to assess what potential risks you are willing to take to achieve what potential benefits. But your decision must be based on all the available medical data, as well as your understanding of what has yet to be determined conclusively.

One of the reasons that women in the past have sometimes felt they have been treated patronizingly by breast surgeons is that they are interacting at a time when it is extremely difficult for almost any human being to behave in an unemotional and dispassionately logical fashion. They have been told not just that they have a malignancy, but a malignancy in an organ that is linked, in our society, to a woman's sexuality. Under the circumstances, it is terribly difficult to appear totally calm and logical. Frequently, in past years, the doctor told the patient what he felt had to be done, without discussing alternatives, and the patient listened and obeyed, without asking questions. It sometimes appeared to physicians that at this time of extreme stress, a patient could not manage to sort out a large amount of complex and not clearly defined data and arrive at a clear-cut conclusion. Fortunately, however, patients are becoming more informed. If you have to arrive at a logical decision in a time of such great stress, it is very helpful to have previously acquired a good understanding of the issues involved.

Since each woman has a one-in-eleven chance of developing breast cancer in her lifetime, and since it is difficult to assimilate information on the success of various therapies at a time when your logic may be overtaken by fear, and since it should be you yourself who make the final decision regarding treatment for your own body, it seems imperative that you think about this issue now, when you are healthy, rational, and unemotional.

CHAPTER VII

Surgery for Breast Cancer

Breast cancer has been a significant problem through the ages; there is historical reference to the disease dating back to 3000–2500 B.C. Unfortunately, modern medicine has just started to catch up. It is only during the last century that medically sophisticated, carefully planned approaches to the surgical therapy of breast cancer have been repeatedly refined, as physicians have learned increasingly more about the biologic behavior of breast cancer.

Several factors must be taken into consideration in attempting to define the optimal surgical procedure for breast cancer in general, and, more important, in selecting the surgical procedure for an individual breast cancer affecting one particular woman.

In determining the proper operation for an individual woman's breast cancer, each of these questions should be considered:

1. Which operation will give the woman the greatest chance to be cured?

2. Which operation will offer the woman the best cosmetic results?

3. What are the woman's priorities? Each woman obviously must be approached as an individual, and her own needs, concerns, and priorities must be considered.

4. Which operation will provide the best functional result? Particularly important is maintaining full function and strength of the arm and shoulder on the affected side.

5. Which operation is associated with the fewest short-term and long-term complications?

Once each of these questions has been answered, the appropriate surgical procedure will become somewhat more apparent. Each tumor must be evaluated in terms of its unique and specific features, as must each patient. Only a doctor who knows your particular medical situation in great detail should make recommendations for your care, based on the size of the tumor, its involvement of lymph nodes, its location, its appearance under the microscope, and its involvement of other structures such as the skin, muscle, chest wall, bone, and distant organs. Your age and general health are also of great significance.

In about 1882, William Halsted, a professor of surgery at the Johns Hopkins Medical School in Baltimore, developed and then subsequently refined the operation that was to prevail for almost the next hundred years as the preferred surgery for the woman with breast cancer: the radical mastectomy. The radical mastectomy involves removal of the breast, the underlying muscles (pectoralis major and pectoralis minor), and the lymph nodes and fatty tissue in the axilla (armpit). At the time when it was conceived and refined, this procedure represented an enormous contribution to women's health and to modern medicine; the radical mastectomy resulted in the cure of breast cancer for hundreds of thousands of women. Unfortunately, because the radical mastectomy includes the removal of the very important pectoralis muscles, it does frequently result in both a significant cosmetic deformity and impaired functioning and weakness of the arm and shoulder on the affected side. The resulting concavity of the chest wall and axilla are often apparent when a woman who has had this surgery wears standard sportswear, a bathing suit, and even some typical daytime and evening wear. This operation may also result in lymphedema (swelling) of the arm.

Yet, because this operation was the first procedure devised that could truly offer a woman a reasonably good chance to be cured of breast cancer, and because the lesser procedures that had been performed earlier were nowhere near so successful, it was many decades before the radical mastectomy was challenged as the optimal surgical procedure. Until 1970, approximately half of the American women who had surgery each year for breast cancer were treated by radical mastectomy rather than by a less aggressive operation, which could provide a better functional and cosmetic result. By 1976, only one-quarter of the American women with breast cancer were being treated by radical mastectomy. This number has continued to decline in the last decade.

Many surgeons feel that there is a role for the radical mastectomy in modern medicine, for a limited group of women who have very specific reasons for requiring this more extensive operative procedure.

One example is a woman whose breast cancer involves the pectoralis muscle: a radical mastectomy might be recommended since if the pectoralis muscle was preserved, tumor would obviously be left in the woman's body.

Although the trend in the last decade has, appropriately,

been away from radical surgery and toward a much more limited surgical approach, one operative procedure that some surgeons feel continues to be a valid approach to the care of the patient with extensive breast cancer removes even more than the radical mastectomy. This operation is called the extended radical mastectomy. In this operation, besides removing the breast, pectoralis major and minor muscles, and axillary fat and nodes, the surgeon may also remove the internal mammary nodes, parasternal nodes (additional nodes that run deep in the middle of the chest), and a portion of the chest wall. This operation may result in considerable concavity of the chest. Now that more is known about the biology of breast cancer and its routes of dissemination, there is more of a tendency to approach extensive disease with surgery plus other modes of therapy rather than to resort to the extended radical mastectomy. Some data, however, do support the extended radical mastectomy as a potentially curative procedure for the woman with extensive disease.

During the 1960s, the radical mastectomy was still considered by many physicians to be the procedure of choice for the woman with breast cancer. So much has been achieved since then. The goal has been to continue to provide women the same opportunity for cure of breast cancer while offering improved cosmetic and functional results. The first, major contribution toward that goal was the trend away from the radical mastectomy and toward the modified radical mastectomy.

The modified radical mastectomy is similar to the radical mastectomy, but less tissue is removed. The major difference between the two operations is that the modified radical mastectomy leaves the pectoralis major muscle intact. (Some surgeons do not remove the pectoralis minor muscle, either.) The pectoralis major muscle is important for

Figures 1–4 This woman was discovered to have breast cancer when she was fifty-nine years old. After counseling, she elected to have removal of the tumor and lymph nodes in the underarm, followed by radiation therapy, rather than to have a mastectomy. An eight-millimeter tumor was thus removed from her

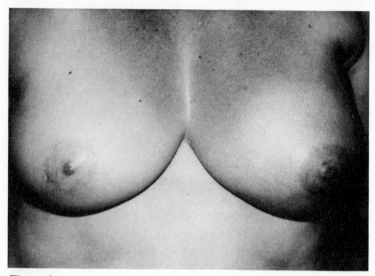

Figure 1

Figure 2

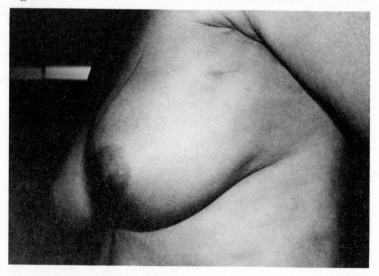

left breast (a small scar is visible in figure 2), as were the lymph nodes in her underarm (none of which contained tumor). Then, she underwent radiation therapy. These photographs were taken six months after she completed therapy, at which time she was healthy and free of tumor. (Photographs courtesy of Dr. Herschel Flax.)

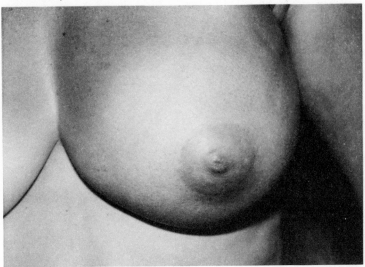

Figure 3

Figure 4

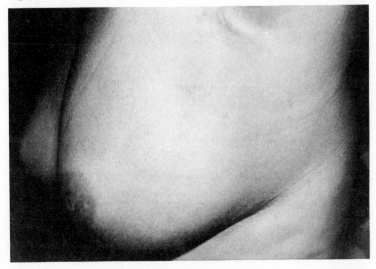

Figures 5–8 This woman was discovered to have breast cancer when she was thirty-nine years old. After counseling, she elected to have the tumor removed and radiation therapy administered, rather than a mastectomy. The tumor was six millimeters in size and was in the upper outer portion of her right breast. She remains free of breast cancer six years after therapy. (Photographs courtesy of Dr. Herschel Flax.)

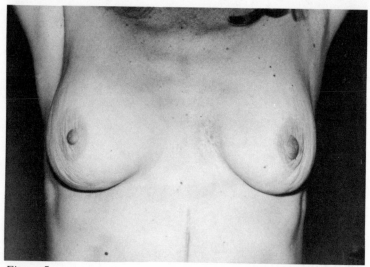

Figure 5
Figure 6

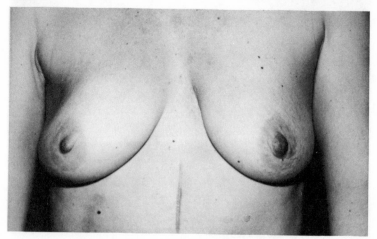

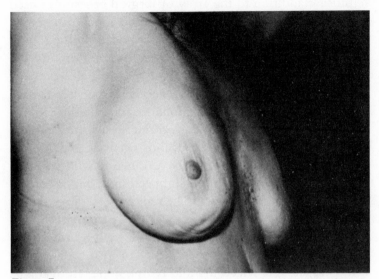

Figure 7
Figure 8

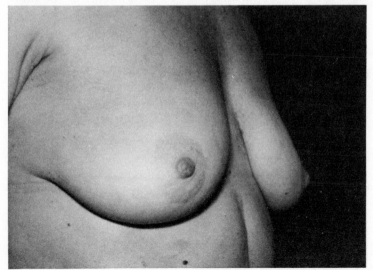

flexing the arm, rotating it, and moving it toward the body. Obviously, an operation that can preserve this muscle while still affording the woman the same chance of cure is a very significant addition to the array of surgical procedures used to cure breast cancer. The cosmetic and functional results are a vast improvement over those provided by the radical mastectomy, and, for most women, the opportunity for cure is the same.

As was discussed in chapter VI, another major step toward improving cosmetic and functional results for the woman with breast cancer without jeopardizing her chances of cure is at present receiving a great deal of attention and appears to be quite promising for many groups of women. This operation is called tylectomy (lumpectomy), and is usually performed in conjunction with the removal of axillary lymph nodes. After the operation the woman is treated with radiation; under certain circumstances she may be advised to undergo chemotherapy as well.

It is hoped that tylectomy and lymph node removal plus radiation therapy will be demonstrated to afford the patient the same opportunity for long-term cure as the more extensive surgical procedures already described, and there is a large body of evidence suggesting that it will. But even this limited procedure does have some drawbacks. A woman with very small breasts, very large breasts, or a very large tumor, as discussed in the last chapter, might end up with significant cosmetic deformity when treated with a lumpectomy and radiation, and might actually have preferable cosmetic results with mastectomy and reconstruction. In addition, the lumpectomy should be done in such a way that all traces of the malignancy are removed, with a margin of healthy tissue around the tumor removed as well. If the pathologist looks at the tissue removed in a lumpectomy and finds tumor at the margin of the excised tissue (indicating a significant possibility that some tumor may still be in the patient's remaining breast tissue), the surgeon may still need to remove the breast. In addition, some women have breast cancer that is multicentric (arising in more than one location). For these women, lumpectomy might serve to remove a malignancy that has originated in one area of the breast, while neglecting a malignant focus arising in another site. Therefore, despite the obvious benefits of lumpectomy in many situations, it is clearly not the procedure of choice for all breast cancers.

The last two decades have certainly witnessed a turn away from more extensive breast cancer surgery. However, under some circumstances a woman might decide that a mastectomy is appropriate, although she does not even have a breast malignancy. One example of this is the prophylactic subcutaneous mastectomy.

In a subcutaneous mastectomy, the breast tissue is removed but the skin overlying the breast is left in place. Then a breast prosthesis (artificial breast) is placed underneath the skin. After this operation the breast appears normal, although the breast tissue has in fact been removed.

It may seem somewhat contradictory to perform a type of mastectomy on a woman who doesn't even have breast cancer, at a time when we are trying to avoid mastectomy even when a woman does have breast cancer. However, subcutaneous mastectomy appears to be an operation with potential validity for certain groups of women. As has been discussed extensively in chapter II, some women are at extremely high risk of developing breast cancer. If a woman has cancer in one breast, there is a significant likelihood that she will ultimately develop cancer in the other breast. Women who have several relatives with breast cancer (such as mother, sister and grandmother) are at extremely high risk. Once a woman develops breast cancer, she obviously becomes at risk to die of the disease. Therefore, a woman with a very high risk of developing breast cancer might elect to have a subcutaneous mastectomy and prosthesis even though she is perfectly healthy, rather than live in fear of developing the disease. Unfortunately, however, a subcutaneous mastectomy does not fully eliminate the possibility of developing a breast cancer, since a small amount of tissue remains when this operation is performed. Therefore, some women choose to have a prophylactic total mastectomy (removal of the entire breast, overlying skin, and nipple).

The decision to have a prophylactic subcutaneous or total mastectomy with the implant of a prosthesis is not made very often, but appears to be most commonly made by women who have already had a cancer in one breast or whose relatives developed breast cancer at a young age, particularly when several close relatives were affected. Obviously, this is a very difficult decision for a woman to make, and one requiring extensive consideration and counseling.

There is one instance in which some breast surgeons feel that a woman should have a mastectomy even though she does not have an invasive breast cancer. This is for a condition called breast carcinoma *in situ*. Breast carcinoma *in situ* is a premalignant condition. However, women with carcinoma *in situ*, especially those in which the carcinoma *in situ* has a certain appearance when viewed under the microscope, are at extremely high risk of developing invasive breast cancer. Some surgeons, therefore, recommend mastectomy even though these women do not have a truly invasive cancer. The use of lumpectomy plus radiation for this problem is under investigation at present, but is still considered experimental; it has not yet been thoroughly evaluated as a treatment for carcinoma *in situ*.

There are many things doctors do not yet know about breast cancer. As discussed, the optimal surgical therapy will vary, depending upon the size of the tumor, whether it involves the lymph nodes, what it looks like under the microscope, its location, whether it involves the chest wall, whether it involves any other structures, and the woman's age and general health. In addition, even when one individual woman with her unique breast cancer seeks an opinion regarding what is the best therapy for her particular tumor, it is not unlikely that she will get two different opinions if she goes to two different doctors.

What, then, should a woman with breast cancer do to assure that the surgery recommended for her is indeed the best choice for her? The answer really is that the woman must be certain that she is informed about the disease. She must listen carefully to her doctor's suggestions and then make sure she fully understands all therapeutic alternatives, including their potential risks and benefits, and the likelihood of cure they entail. There are some answers the doctor cannot provide, because, as we've seen, some information still remains unknown. However, the woman who requires surgery for breast cancer must make certain that to the extent that the information is available, she understands all that is known about the appropriate therapeutic options that exist for her particular situation. Only then can she make a rational, informed decision.

CHAPTER VIII

Radiation Therapy

The role of radiation therapy in the treatment of breast cancer has changed considerably in recent years. In the past, the technique was used almost exclusively for patients who had advanced disease. As chemotherapy has developed into a more effective method of treatment, radiation therapy has been used less frequently postoperatively for women with advanced disease, since for many of these women chemotherapy has taken its place. However, radiation therapy has now come to play an ever-increasing role in the treatment of breast cancers that are detected early.

As was discussed in chapter VI, a growing body of scientific evidence suggests that women with early breast cancer may be cured just as readily if treated by removal of the tumor and lymph nodes from the underarm, followed by postoperative radiation, as she would be if treated by mastectomy. Because women who have been treated for breast cancer may develop a recurrence of the disease as long as twenty years after the tumor was originally treated, and since the studies that evaluate radiation as primary therapy for breast cancer have not yet been ongoing for twenty years, it is impossible to say that a woman treated without mastectomy will definitely have the same chance of being cured as she would have if her breast had been removed. However, many physicians, myself included, do believe that when these studies have been extended for the full twenty years, they will confirm the treatment of breast cancer without mastectomy as excellent therapy, providing the same rate of cure, usually with no physical disfigurement and certainly with much less psychological trauma. In any event, even though no guarantees can yet be given, large numbers of women have elected to be treated by lumpectomy, lymph node removal, and radiation therapy, preserving the breast.

After the lumpectomy and lymph node removal have been completed, the breast tissue and surgical scar are allowed to heal. Then, within the next few weeks, radiation therapy begins. At the woman's first visit with the radiation therapist, the doctor will examine her breasts and determine a "treatment plan." This means deciding how the radiation should be given, what the boundaries of the tissue to be irradiated should be, and how many treatments will be required. The doctor will then mark the woman's skin with red ink to outline the area that is to be treated with radiation. This ink will stay on for the entire duration of the treatment; it fades slowly over time and does not wash away in the shower. The markings are very important: they are used to identify the exact boundaries for the treatment, so that each day when a patient receives her radiation, the technician will be able to identify and irradiate exactly the same tissue.

The room in which the radiation is administered may seem somewhat eerie to the patient at first. It is usually large and is dominated by an enormous machine from which the radiation emanates. The patient lies on a long metal table under this machine, and the radiation technician positions her so that she will receive the radiation in the correct spot. The technician will then leave the room so that he or she is not exposed to the effects of radiation. There is an intercom so that the patient can easily communicate with the technician, and a closed-circuit television so that the technician can make certain the patient does not move while receiving her treatment, since this would cause the beam of radiation to be directed at the wrong tissue. Once everything is in place, the technician turns on the switch and the radiation emanates from the machine. Although every patient's radiation regimen may be a bit different, each treatment lasts about two minutes.

For the first few treatments, many patients feel strange, lying alone in a room under an enormous machine that is emitting radiation. However, most people get used to it after a few days.

Treatments are usually delivered in this fashion five days a week for approximately five weeks. Following that, some women may receive a few additional weeks of localized therapy, which is given in a similar fashion but in which a much smaller amount of tissue is irradiated, or the radiation therapist may recommend an iridium implant. The decision whether to use electrons or an iridium implant will depend in part upon what is available at the particular hospital or radiation-treatment facility, as well as on the location of the cancer and the size of the breast. Both methods seem to be equally beneficial in the treatment of primary breast cancer following lumpectomy.

To undergo an iridium implant, a woman must be admitted to the hospital. The procedure is usually performed in an operating room, with the woman under general anesthesia. Needles are placed in the breast to serve as guides for the placement of plastic tubes, somewhat similar to the way a needle and thread are used in sewing. Once the plastic tubes are in place in the breast tissue, the needles are removed, and then the patient is awakened and taken back to her room. It is here that the radioactive material (iridium) is put into the plastic tubes in her breast, so that the number of hospital personnel exposed to the radiation can be minimized. After about two days, the iridium and the plastic tubes are removed.

The patient may have some mild discomfort when the iridium and plastic tubes are in place, but this can be easily alleviated with medication. During the two-day period, the patient will be in a private room. She is not confined to the bed; she can sit in a chair or walk around the room. She can have visitors, though not children or pregnant women, but it is advised that visitors stay at least six feet away from the patient and not remain in the room for more than an hour on any given day, so that their exposure to the radiation can be limited. The amount of radiation visitors receive if they follow this plan is not thought to represent any threat to their health.

Most women who are treated for their early breast cancer primarily by radiation therapy do not experience serious side effects, but in some women they may occur. These may include local itching, swelling, or skin changes in the area being radiated. Also, patients occasionally complain of fatigue. The radiation therapist will discuss all the potential side effects with the patient before treatment is begun.

Radiation may alter the appearance, consistency, texture, and sensitivity of the breast. Occasionally, the breast may appear somewhat pulled and have a tougher consistency, and a small percentage of women are not satisfied with the end result. Also, in a small number of women the radiation fails to eliminate the disease, so that they may still require a mastectomy. Other possible but uncommon side effects include the potential for rib fracture, radiation-induced pneumonia, or pericardial effusion (fluid surrounding the heart). These problems may occur because the ribs, lungs, and heart are close to the breast, and they

77

therefore unavoidably receive some radiation when the breast is being treated. There may also be a decrease in the number of white blood cells (the cells that ward off infection) or platelets (which help the blood to clot). In general, however, women who are treated for breast cancer by primary radiation therapy have excellent cosmetic results and minimal significant side effects.

Although radiation therapy has become such an important mode of treatment for the woman whose breast cancer is diagnosed early, we must remember that it can also be extremely helpful to the woman who has an advanced primary tumor or to the woman who has metastatic breast cancer.

Two decades ago, a much larger proportion of women who had a mastectomy received radiation therapy after their surgery. The use of radiation therapy diminished as the benefits of post-mastectomy chemotherapy became apparent, but radiation therapy following mastectomy still offers help to some subgroups of women. There is, however, controversy over precisely which women should receive it.

Women who have locally advanced breast cancer that is treated by aggressive surgery are still at considerable risk of developing a recurrence of the malignancy, both on the chest wall and at distant sites, such as in the bone or the abdomen. Either chemotherapy or hormonal therapy (see chapter IX) is usually used in such cases in an attempt to prevent or delay the recurrence of the cancer. Treating such a patient with radiation therapy postoperatively does not improve her chances of cure, but it will considerably diminish the likelihood that her breast cancer will recur locally, in the area treated with postoperative radiation therapy. Advocates of postoperative radiation feel that this can be of considerable benefit to the patient. They feel that since a local recurrence frequently happens before distant metastases appear, postoperative radiation may provide the woman with a longer interval of good health before recurrent cancer develops. On the other hand, those who are not strong supporters of postmastectomy radiation therapy feel that if a recurrence does develop locally, it can usually be effectively treated with radiation at that time, and that withholding such therapy unless a local recurrence occurs may spare many women the need for local radiation therapy.

The decision as to precisely which women should receive postmastectomy radiation therapy in an attempt to prevent local recurrence of the cancer remains somewhat controversial. If it is going to be used, it should be for those women who are at high risk of developing a recurrence on their chest wall. This may include women whose tumor is in blood vessels, involves a large proportion of the lymph nodes, has grown through the capsule of a lymph node, is very large, or is located in the inner portion of the breast, and clearly includes women whose tumor has extended to the margin of surgical resection (the tumor extends all the way to the line where the surgeon made the incision). Not all doctors would employ postoperative radiation for each of the aforementioned problems; some difference of opinion remains.

Almost all women who are at high risk of developing a recurrence on the chest wall following mastectomy are also at risk of developing distant metastases. Therefore, a woman may be advised to have both chemotherapy and radiation therapy postoperatively, the radiation to prevent the recurrence of tumor on the chest wall, the chemotherapy to destroy any tumor cells present in the body, to avoid the return of malignancy. This combination of radiation and chemotherapy may be delivered in what is referred to as the "sandwich technique." Following surgery, the patient receives some chemotherapy; she is then treated with radiation; then the chemotherapy is resumed. The radiation therapy is thus tucked in the middle, with chemotherapy both before and after it.

For women who have very advanced breast cancer, therapy that combines radiation, chemotherapy, and surgery may be advised. Some cancers are clearly so extensive that surgery could not remove all the local tumor. Some of these women will be treated by very extensive radiation and chemotherapy without surgery. In other situations, the addition of surgery may be thought to reduce the chance of immediate local problems, and it may, therefore, be included in the treatment regimen.

We doctors hope that the great degree of awareness of their bodies that many women have now acquired will make them more likely to perform breast self-examination and be screened for the early detection of breast cancer, so that we will see fewer and fewer women with incurable advanced disease.

Besides being used in an attempt to prevent the return of breast cancer, radiation therapy may also be employed should a recurrence develop. A large proportion of women with recurrent breast cancer will be advised to have treatment with chemotherapy or hormones. However, if a localized area of tumor is producing a problem, radiation therapy may be quite helpful. It has an effect on tumor only in the area in which the radiation beam is directed, whereas hormones and chemotherapy are referred to as "systemic therapy" because they circulate through the system and can exert their beneficial effect in most areas of the body. Therefore, radiation can be utilized to treat a problem in a specific location. However, for women with recurrent breast cancer, if radiation is given it is usually in conjunction with systemic therapy, since once recurrent disease has been identified in one area of the body, the presence of tumor cells in other areas as well is a strong possibility. The radiation exerts its effect on the local problem while the chemotherapy destroys occult (hidden) or obvious malignant cells elsewhere in the body.

There are several circumstances in which radiation therapy would be extremely useful in treating recurrent breast cancer. One such instance is when breast cancer has metastasized to the bone. Bone metastases can be quite painful, and irradiating the area where they have occurred can often remove this pain. Tumor that metastasizes to a weight-bearing site in the bone may present significant problems. For instance, the femur is the bone of the thigh, and the "head" of the femur is the part of the bone that articulates with the hip joint. Metastases to the femur may occur and, if untreated or unresponsive to treatment, may result in a fracture, which could significantly impair the woman's mobility. Irradiation of such a metastasis may prevent this. For some women, hip pinning (the placement of a piece of metal in the bone) may be necessary as well.

If cancer recurs on the chest wall, this can be eliminated in approximately fifty percent of cases with radiation therapy—as long as the woman has not already received radiation to the area. The same area usually cannot be irradiated twice, since doing so might result in excessive destruction of normal tissue or in infection. However, for the woman who has not had prior chest-wall irradiation, the technique is an excellent method of eradicating this type of local recurrence.

Occasionally, a woman whose breast cancer has metastasized to the lung will develop pneumonia beyond the tumor or will cough up blood because of the lesion. The physician may, therefore, decide to irradiate a focal region (small area) of the lung. We must realize, though, that the radiation in such circumstances is directed at controlling the local problem; it is almost never able to cure the patient fully of her malignancy.

If breast cancer has metastasized to the region of the spinal cord, this may produce paralysis. Radiation to the area may shrink the tumor enough to restore muscular function. Metastases to the liver may produce severe pain if the capsule (outer covering) of the liver is stretched by the tumor. Irradiating the affected portion may alleviate the pain.

When a woman develops recurrent breast cancer in such crucial areas as the spinal cord, lung, or liver, radiation therapy to these areas will not cure her of metastatic disease. What it can do is to shrink the tumor in the crucial area of concern to avoid a serious problem (such as paralysis from tumor compressing the spinal cord). Radiation in these circumstances is almost always used in conjunction with chemotherapy or hormonal therapy, in the hope that the systemic therapy will prolong the patient's life by eliminating as many tumor cells as possible throughout the body. Since, as discussed, the radiation destroys only cells in the path of its beam, it will be of benefit in treating the acute problem but will not destroy tumor cells elsewhere.

In summary, radiation is a very important treatment method for patients who have breast cancer. For women who have an early stage of the disease, it can be used to eradicate the tumor, so that mastectomy can be avoided. For women who have advanced primary breast cancer, it can be used after a mastectomy to reduce the chance of recurrent disease on the chest wall. For the patient who has a primary breast cancer that is so advanced that it cannot be removed, mastectomy may be omitted and only radiation plus chemotherapy used to control the disease. When recurrent breast cancer is present, radiation can frequently shrink an isolated focus of disease and alleviate serious symptomatology. Radiation therapy can be employed in so many different ways to control the pain, eradicate a focus of disease, or save the life of a woman with breast cancer.

CHAPTER IX

Chemotherapy, Hormonal Therapy, and Interferon Therapy

Chemotherapy is of enormous potential benefit to the woman who has breast cancer. Unfortunately, many people regard chemotherapy as the treatment of last resort, and consider its use to be synonymous with imminent disaster. Although this may be true with a few other types of malignancies, it is for the most part a false assumption in the case of women with breast cancer. The benefits of chemotherapy for these women have been extensively evaluated and our capacity to use these drugs to great advantage has been further defined and refined. Many studies to evaluate more fully the role of chemotherapy for the woman who has been treated for breast cancer are in progress now; our knowledge grows daily.

We have learned so much about the benefits of chemotherapy for the woman with breast cancer that it is at present used not only to control the spread of tumor in women who are known to have recurrent disease, but also to prevent the return of cancer in women who have completed their primary cancer therapy and have no evidence of disease. Chemotherapy for breast cancer appears to have enormous potential benefit when used for either of these two reasons.

I feel it is important that the very positive medical benefits chemotherapy can offer not be diminished by its pejorative connotation, and I believe that doctors, patients, and the general public should work in concert to achieve this goal. How can this happen? When a woman's physician recommends that she have chemotherapy, it is important that all the potential benefits, risks, and alternatives are fully discussed. If a woman understands why chemotherapy has been recommended in her particular circumstance, and all the possible beneficial effects it can have (including preventing her from ever developing a recurrence of the malignancy, and curing her fully of the disease), she is more likely to feel positively about its use, and thus be better able to accept any of the side effects she may experience.

Besides making sure that the notion that chemotherapy means impending disaster is dispelled for the patient herself, we must also convince her family and friends. Again, the only way to achieve this is through education. If a woman receiving chemotherapy understands all of the potential positive effects this may have for her, but her family and friends are behaving anxiously and giving her signals that they believe the situation is ominous, this will certainly make it difficult for her to respond positively to her therapy, to face her future with hope and calm.

As will be discussed later in this chapter, chemotherapy is not without potential side effects and discomfort. However, I have found that patients who understand all the potential positive effects the treatment may offer them are usually quite willing to tolerate the side effects. In fact, it often seems to me that a woman who is optimistic about all the positive things chemotherapy can do for her is less likely to be bothered by side effects or discomforts from the drugs.

WHAT IS CHEMOTHERAPY AND HOW DOES IT WORK?

Chemotherapy is treatment by drugs, and for women with breast cancer these drugs are used to destroy tumor cells. Some forms of chemotherapy can be taken in pills, some are injected into the muscle, and some are injected into the vein.

There are dozens of types of chemotherapeutic drugs being employed to treat malignancies at present. Of all these, only certain ones will be useful to treat any particular type of malignancy. It is fortunate that many different drugs are active in destroying breast cancer cells. These drugs are grouped according to their mechanisms of action (the ways the drugs work to destroy tumor cells). Some of the useful types of drugs employed in treating breast cancer include:

ALKYLATING AGENTS
These drugs prevent tumor cells from dividing. They do this by cross-linking the two strands of the DNA, which are the cell's building blocks. The other components of the tumor cell, particularly its RNA and protein, will continue to be produced, growth will become unbalanced, and the tumor cell will die. Some examples of alkylating agents that have been shown to be useful for women with breast cancer include:

Chlorambucil (Leukeran)

Cyclophosphamide (Cytoxan)

Melphalan (Alkeran)

Nitrogen mustard (Mustargen)

Triethylenethiophosphoramide (Thiotepa)

ANTIMETABOLITES

These chemotherapeutic agents work by interfering with the building blocks required to make DNA and RNA. Without these building blocks, the tumor cells are unable to make DNA or RNA, and they die. Examples of antimetabolites used to treat breast cancer include:

Amethopterin (Methotrexate)

5-Fluorouracil (5-FU)

ANTIBIOTICS

These have some similarity to the antibiotics used to treat infections, but they destroy tumor cells rather than bacteria. One of the most effective chemotherapeutic agents employed to eradicate breast cancer (Adriamycin) is included in this group of antineoplastic antibiotics (antibiotics that destroy tumor cells). Antibiotics that have been shown to be useful in the treatment of breast cancer include:

Doxorubicin (Adriamycin)

Mutamycin (Mitomycin C)

PLANT ALKALOIDS

These chemotherapeutic agents, derived from the periwinkle plant, work by inhibiting mitosis (cell division), so that the tumor cells are unable to divide. Examples of plant alkaloids used to treat breast cancer include:

Vincristine (Oncovin)

Vinblastine (Velban)

MISCELLANEOUS AGENTS
Some antineoplastic agents cannot be categorized in any of the previous four groups, but are quite effective. One that might be used in treating breast cancer is:

Hydroxyurea (Hydrea)

DOES CHEMOTHERAPY HAVE SIDE EFFECTS?

Chemotherapy has many potential positive effects for the woman with breast cancer. It can help to prevent the recurrence of cancer when used prophylactically (as extra prevention) for the woman whose tumor appears to have been eradicated by surgery. If cancer does recur, chemotherapy can eradicate the tumor or slow its growth.

Chemotherapy is able to achieve its beneficial effects by destroying cells. All cells, both healthy and malignant, are at risk of being affected by the process, but since tumor cells are usually dividing more rapidly than normal cells, they are more likely to be destroyed by chemotherapy. In addition, normal cells seem better able to withstand the effects of chemotherapy, undergo repair, and return to efficient functioning. Therefore, although chemotherapy is able to exert an influence upon all cells, thus producing many "side effects" through its influence on normal cells, it fortunately exerts a more profound destructive effect on malignant cells. It is essential, however, that before receiving chemotherapy the patient be fully informed by her doctor regarding all potential side effects of the medications.

Some of the side effects are merely annoying. Others can cause quite a bit of discomfort. For these types of problems, I find that if the patient understands why she is receiving chemotherapy and what its potential benefits are, the irritants become less distressing and even less noticeable to her. But some forms of side effects, though they may not even be apparent to the patient, have the potential to cause serious consequences. Since these problems are usually not noticed by the patient unless they have already produced some damage, they are monitored quite carefully by her doctor.

What follows is a description of some of the more common side effects that can be produced by chemotherapy.

NAUSEA AND VOMITING
Chemotherapy often triggers the vomiting centers in the brain and may produce extreme nausea and vomiting. For women being treated with drugs that are known to produce these problems, medication is frequently administered to reduce the side effects. Fortunately, some new drugs introduced recently are quite effective in reducing this uncomfortable problem.

GASTROINTESTINAL DISTRESS
The cells that line the intestines normally divide very rapidly. Since many of the chemotherapeutic agents are effective because they interfere with cell division, the cells of the intestines are likely to be affected by the drugs.

HAIR LOSS
This may be particularly distressing, since it may be difficult for a woman to reassure herself of her excellent progress and to respond positively to her therapy while she is

losing her hair. Many of the drugs that are the most effective in treating breast cancer are known to produce significant hair loss. As is the case with the cells that line the bowel, hair follicles grow very rapidly, and cells that are active are the ones most likely to be susceptible to the effects of chemotherapy.

Fortunately, many lovely wigs are available. Obviously, almost all women feel more attractive with their own hair than with a wig, which they feel compelled to wear. However, I have seen women who actually look more attractive in the stylish wigs they were obliged to buy because of their chemotherapy than they looked with their own hair.

If a woman is going to be receiving chemotherapy that is known to produce hair loss, it may be worthwhile for her to go shopping for a wig before she has actually lost any hair. She can then shop at her leisure until she finds a style that pleases her and gives her a positive feeling about herself. Women who wait until they have lost their hair to purchase a wig may already feel unattractive and distressed and will never be as pleased with the wig as they would have been if they had purchased it earlier.

In some instances, a woman's insurance company may pay for her wig if it is prescribed by her physician and she needs it because of her chemotherapy. A woman who will be undergoing chemotherapy that is expected to result in hair loss should discuss this with her doctor and with her insurance company.

It is encouraging for women to know that this hair loss is not permanent. The hair will begin to grow back once chemotherapy has been terminated.

FATIGUE, LETHARGY, AND DEPRESSION

Many people who are undergoing chemotherapy have these complaints, because of their psychological reaction to the malignancy itself as well as the effects of chemotherapy. Even for the woman whose outlook and approach to her malignancy are most optimistic, chemotherapy is frequently quite fatiguing; such effects are often compounded when a woman is depressed about the illness itself.

BONE MARROW SUPPRESSION

White blood cells, platelets, and red blood cells are produced in the bone marrow. Because the rate of production of white blood cells (which assist in preventing infection) and platelets (which are important components in helping the blood to clot) is very rapid, the white blood cell and platelet production is frequently very sensitive to chemotherapy. Red blood cells survive in the body for a longer time and are therefore usually less severely affected.

When the number of white blood cells becomes very low, the patient may have great difficulty warding off infection. When the platelet count becomes very low, the patient may suddenly begin to bleed, internally or externally. Therefore, when a woman is receiving chemotherapy, her physician will be monitoring her white blood cell count, platelet count, and red blood cell count. If the doctor is concerned that the counts are becoming too low, chemotherapy will be temporarily withheld until the bone marrow has an opportunity to repair itself and starts to produce white blood cells and platelets in adequate numbers once more.

Occasionally, the white blood cell count becomes so low that the woman develops a fever and requires hospitalization and antibiotics. If the number of white cells becomes extremely low, the woman may be placed in reverse isolation for a few days. This means that everyone who comes in contact with her must wear a gown, mask, and gloves to avoid spreading germs to her, since her body will usually be unable to ward off infection.

A patient may require a platelet transfusion if the number of platelets has been reduced to such a small number that she is in danger of spontaneous bleeding. Blood transfusions may be given if the chemotherapy has caused the woman to become severely anemic (having a lowered red blood cell count).

Usually, however, unless the counts become extremely low and the patient develops problems, a woman receiving chemotherapy is not even aware that her bone marrow is being suppressed.

NEUROLOGIC CHANGES

Certain of the chemotherapeutic agents can produce muscle weakness and abnormal neural sensations. If these become severe, the drug that is thought to be producing the problem may have to be withheld.

STOMATITIS (MOUTH ULCERATION)

Some of the drugs used in the treatment of breast cancer may produce sores in the mouth. Chemotherapy is usually temporarily withheld when this occurs, since the presence of such sores may be an indication that there are also simultaneous ulcerations in other areas of the gastrointestinal tract, such as the bowel.

CYSTITIS

Bladder inflammation, occasionally causing bleeding from the lining of the bladder resulting in blood in the urine, may be caused by Cytoxan chemotherapy.

SKIN CHANGES

Rashes, deepening of pigment, and desquamation (shedding) of superficial skin may be caused by some of the chemotherapeutic agents.

CARDIAC (HEART) TOXICITY

This potentially serious problem can occur predominantly from the use of Adriamycin. Since Adriamycin is a very important drug for the treatment of breast cancer and is thought by some investigators to possibly be the best single drug available, it will probably continue to be used for many women. Doctors are cautious when administering this drug, constantly alert to any changes suggesting weakness of the heart muscle, which would indicate that they must discontinue the use of Adriamycin.

In addition, doctors are willing to use no more than a specified maximum amount of Adriamycin for any patient, since above that dose the likelihood of heart-muscle damage increases greatly.

LIVER TOXICITY

Some forms of chemotherapy may damage the liver. This effect is usually transient and frequently improves spontaneously if chemotherapy is temporarily withheld.

MISCELLANEOUS SIDE EFFECTS

Other potential risks of chemotherapy include allergic reactions, lung damage, hearing loss, and impaired kidney function.

Although chemotherapy obviously carries serious risks, most women do not experience life-threatening complications, and the potential benefits for the woman with breast cancer can be enormous. It is essential that before being treated with chemotherapy a woman discuss fully with her doctor all the possible risks and benefits given her particular situation, since the pattern varies considerably from patient to patient.

UNDER WHAT CIRCUMSTANCES MIGHT A PHYSICIAN RECOMMEND CHEMOTHERAPY TO A BREAST-CANCER PATIENT?

The initial treatment for breast cancer almost always involves surgery or radiation therapy, and sometimes both are employed. In the past, hormonal therapy and chemotherapy were used only for very advanced primary tumors, or when a woman developed recurrent disease. During the past one and a half decades, data have emerged that suggest that for some women chemotherapy can also be used to prevent or delay the recurrence of breast cancer.

WHAT IS ADJUVANT CHEMOTHERAPY FOR BREAST CANCER AND HOW IS IT USED?

If a woman has completed her primary therapy for breast cancer and is receiving chemotherapy in an attempt to prevent or delay the tumor's recurrence, that is called "adjuvant therapy." During the 1970s, information began to appear in the medical literature that suggested that adjuvant chemotherapy might help reduce the chance that a woman who had been treated for breast cancer would develop recurrent disease in the future. This is a very important problem to be able to address: despite chemotherapy's possible side effects, if we can increase the likelihood that a woman who has been treated for breast cancer can be cured or can live longer without developing recurrent disease, we must find a way to offer such treatment.

Adjuvant chemotherapy appears to be potentially beneficial for many groups of women. If a woman has breast cancer that has spread to her lymph nodes, then, even though the surgeon has removed all identifiable tumor, there is some chance that a few cells may also have metastasized elsewhere in the body, although such cells would not be apparent to the physician or to the patient on any studies that could be performed. For women who are at high risk of micrometastases (very small metastases), chemotherapy given shortly after the initial therapy has been completed may be able either to increase the chance of cure or to increase the interval of time in which the woman remains free of disease.

Although a large amount of research has been performed by hundreds of scientists throughout the world, many questions remain to be answered—and dozens of studies are now under way to answer them. Some of the variables that appear to be important in assessing the likelihood that any individual woman will benefit from a particular adjuvant therapy include whether the woman has gone through menopause and how many nodes contain metastatic tumor. Premenopausal women (those who have not yet had menopause) who have breast cancer that has metastasized to lymph nodes are likely to benefit from adjuvant chemotherapy. If a postmenopausal woman has breast cancer that has metastasized to the nodes, and her tumor contains estrogen receptors, she is more likely to benefit from adjuvant hormonal therapy than by chemotherapy. If she is postmenopausal, has tumor that has metastasized to lymph nodes, but does not have sufficient estrogen receptors in the tumor, she is more likely to benefit from chemotherapy.

More information is constantly being evaluated to answer such questions as whether women who have breast cancer with negative nodes (nodes free of tumor) might benefit from adjuvant chemotherapy, what is the optimal adjuvant therapy given any individual woman's particular circumstances, and how much benefit adjuvant chemotherapy can offer to women when more than ten lymph nodes contain metastatic tumor.

Therefore, only a woman's doctor can really advise her as to what type of adjuvant therapy, if any, would be appropriate given her particular situation. Dr. Gianni Bonadonna, who has contributed extensively to our knowledge about adjuvant chemotherapy for women with breast cancer, has concluded that many patients with primary breast cancer do have micrometastases that cannot be located and surgically eradicated and that the only possibility for preventing or delaying the recurrence of the tumor is with effective systemic therapy.

Any woman who is being treated for breast cancer must understand that adjuvant chemotherapy is chemotherapy given at the completion of primary therapy in the hope of preventing recurrent breast cancer or delaying the onset of recurrence. Each patient should have a thorough discussion with her physician regarding the potential benefits and risks, given the exact nature of her situation, since the benefits of adjuvant chemotherapy, and even what constitutes the best therapy, may vary depending upon the specifics of the woman's situation.

WHEN IS CHEMOTHERAPY HELPFUL IN TREATING RECURRENT BREAST CANCER AND WHEN WOULD HORMONAL THERAPY BE USED INSTEAD?

Since 1969, when Dr. Richard Cooper, a physician from Buffalo, New York, noted for his contributions to our knowledge of chemotherapy for breast cancer, reported excellent results using a regimen of five drugs in combination to treat recurrent breast cancer, there has been extensive research and some enthusiasm for the beneficial effects that combination chemotherapy can have in the treatment of women with recurrent disease. The drugs Dr. Cooper used were Cyclophosphamide, Methotrexate, 5-Fluorouracil, Vincristine, and Prednisone. Physicians call this regimen CMFVP. Although a wide variety of chemotherapeutic regimens continue to be evaluated, one of the common chemotherapy combinations used at present is Cyclophosphamide, Methotrexate, and 5-Fluorouracil. Adriamycin is also extremely effective for breast cancer patients, and is commonly used.

When a woman develops recurrent breast cancer, chemotherapy is not necessarily the treatment of choice. As will be described in the next section, for many women, particularly those whose tumors have a significant amount of estrogen receptors, hormonal therapy may be a more appropriate alternative. A doctor would be more likely to recommend chemotherapy for the woman with recurrent breast cancer under the following circumstances: (1) if the tumor was negative for estrogen receptors, (2) if the woman had failed to respond to previous hormonal therapy, (3) after two hormonal approaches had been used (a relapse following a positive response), or (4) if the tumor is rapidly progressing.

Some women will have a completely successful response to chemotherapy, with all evidence of recurrent breast cancer disappearing. For many other women, chemotherapy will cause a regression of tumor or at least keep the disease from progressing for a while. Although the ideal is obviously for chemotherapy to result in a complete disappearance of disease, it is also an important function of drugs to keep a woman more comfortable and temporarily free from progressive disease.

WHAT IS THE SIGNIFICANCE OF ESTROGEN RECEPTORS?

An estrogen receptor is a substance that binds to and transports estrogen, thereby enabling it to exert its effects on a given cell. The presence and quantity of estrogen receptors and progesterone receptors can be measured in breast cancer tissue that has been surgically removed. This information is important for two reasons, one relating to prognosis and the other to subsequent therapy.

The presence of significant quantities of estrogen receptors and progesterone receptors in a breast cancer is associated with much better cure rates and longer intervals without recurrent disease than would be expected under the same clinical circumstances when the tumor did not contain significant quantities of receptors. For instance, if two women of the same age had breast cancers identical in size, location, and the number of lymph nodes containing metastatic tumor, but one woman's tumor was positive for estrogen receptors and the other's was not, their prognoses would not be the same. Even if all other factors were identical, the woman whose tumor had a significant quantity of estrogen receptors would have a better prognosis.

Knowledge of whether a breast cancer contains receptors will also serve as a guide for subsequent therapy, if any is needed. For women who have advanced or recurrent cancer requiring systemic therapy, it is important to know whether receptors are present in significant quantities: if they are not, a woman is unlikely to respond to hormonal therapy, in which case chemotherapy would be chosen immediately. Therefore, knowing the receptor status of a tumor could save valuable time and prevent the use of hormonal therapy in a situation in which it is highly unlikely to be effective.

If a breast cancer does not have a significant quantity of estrogen receptors or progesterone receptors, there is less than a ten-percent chance that the woman will have a good response to hormonal therapy. If the tumor contains a significant amount of estrogen receptors but not progesterone receptors, there is approximately a thirty-percent chance that hormonal therapy will produce a response. A tumor that has a significant number of progesterone receptors without estrogen receptors is a very unlikely occurrence, but thirty-five to fifty percent of women who have such rare tumors will respond to hormonal therapy. Of patients whose tumors contain significant quantities of both estrogen receptors and progesterone receptors, seventy to eighty percent will respond to hormonal therapy.

Thus knowledge of a tumor's receptor status will give the physician a good idea as to whether hormonal therapy would be likely to result in tumor regression. For patients with receptor-positive tumors, hormonal therapy would be likely to be as effective as chemotherapy while producing fewer side effects.

WHAT IS HORMONAL THERAPY AND WHEN IS IT USEFUL IN TREATING RECURRENT BREAST CANCER?

During the last two decades, there have been major advances in the development of chemotherapy and in its use in the treatment of malignancy. Before that time, the only effective systemic treatment of breast cancer was hormonal therapy. As chemotherapy came to be used more frequently, hormonal-therapy use decreased somewhat.

It has been well studied and documented that hormonal therapy can control recurrent breast cancer and produce long remissions from the disease. Effective hormonal therapies with fewer side effects have been developed, and the use of both hormonal therapy and chemotherapy is now viewed with an enlightened perspective, based on the excellent prospects for beneficial application of each method. Some situations clearly warrant hormonal therapy, in others the indication for chemotherapy is clear-cut, and in some situations either therapy might be appropriate.

At present, many doctors would treat a woman who has recurrent breast cancer with hormonal therapy rather than chemotherapy if her tumor had an adequate level of hormone receptors and if the location and extent of the tumor recurrence did not pose an immediate threat to her. Since it may take as long as several months to determine whether hormonal therapy is having a significant effect on a woman's tumor, the treatment cannot be used when an immediate response is important, such as when the tumor is impairing the function of a vital organ.

The major decision that the doctor treating a woman who has recurrent breast cancer must make is whether she is likely to benefit from hormonal therapy, or whether she should be treated with chemotherapy. Once that has been determined (mostly on the basis of the levels of hormone receptors and the acuteness of the problem), the appropriate choice becomes relatively clear-cut.

If the woman is premenopausal and hormonal therapy is to be undertaken, the hormone therapy the physician may suggest is oöphorectomy (removal of the ovaries), since this will delete a major source of estrogen production. Although this is a relatively simple and uncomplicated operation, the approach favored by doctors in Europe is radiation ablation—radiation therapy to the ovaries until they no longer function. This works somewhat more slowly than surgical removal. Also, women who have breast cancer are at a higher risk than other women are to develop subsequent ovarian cancer, and it may be preferable for them to have their ovaries removed rather than be irradiated. If the premenopausal woman with recurrent breast cancer is to be treated hormonally but is a poor candidate for surgical or radiation ablation of ovarian function, she may be treated with a medication called Tamoxifen, an antiestrogen, which competes with estrogen for binding with the receptor. Tamoxifen will bind with the receptor, thus interfering with the capability of estrogen to do so.

Women who have started to go through menopause or completed menopause and have recurrent breast cancer that is to be treated hormonally are also given Tamoxifen.

Treatment with Tamoxifen is usually continued as long as the woman benefits from therapy. When a woman is treated with the drug, her doctor should monitor her calcium levels, since one potential side effect of Tamoxifen can be to raise the serum calcium too high. If the calcium level becomes extremely high, kidney failure, abnormal heart rhythms, or coma can result. Another rare side effect of

Tamoxifen may be that the tumor actually flares, causing pain at a site of tumor spread. It is important, therefore, that the woman be carefully evaluated by her physician.

If a woman with breast cancer has benefited from one type of hormonal therapy but her tumor subsequently advances, there is a good possibility that she will also derive benefit from another type of hormonal therapy. As is true when making the initial decision to use hormonal treatment, this can only be done when the location or extent of the tumor does not make immediate response to therapy essential.

If the primary hormonal treatment had been removal of ovarian function (either surgically or by radiation), then the secondary hormonal therapy would usually employ Tamoxifen. If the primary hormonal therapy had been Tamoxifen, secondary hormonal therapy would usually be either Megestrol Acetate or Aminoglutethimide plus Hydrocortisone.

Aminoglutethimide exerts its effects by impairing the function of the adrenal gland, a vital regulatory organ of the body, preventing the adrenal gland's conversion of cholesterol to pregnenolone and inhibiting the conversion of androgen to estrogen by blocking a certain mechanism called the "aromatase system." Although this all sounds complex, what it essentially means is that Aminoglutethimide alters the hormonal balance. The development of Aminoglutethimide has represented a major advance in the treatment of women with breast cancer, since before it was available women had to undergo surgical removal of their adrenal glands to achieve the same effect. This is a major operative procedure, and therefore is much more risky than treatment with Aminoglutethimide. People who are treated with Aminoglutethimide must simultaneously receive Hydrocortisone so that they do not develop the very serious symptoms of adrenal insufficiency.

Although Aminoglutethimide produces more significant side effects than Tamoxifen, most patients do tolerate this therapy quite well. The major side effects that may commonly occur are some tiredness, a drug rash, and dizziness, but these can usually be managed by adjusting the doses of the Hydrocortisone and the Aminoglutethimide.

Other hormones that have been used to treat recurrent breast cancer include Diethylstilbestrol (DES), Fluoxymesterone (an androgen), and Medroxyprogesterone acetate (a progestational agent).

It is clear that for appropriately selected patients who have recurrent or advanced breast cancer, hormonal therapy can be extremely effective in producing a remission.

Hormonal therapy may also be a good adjuvant therapy in certain situations. Postmenopausal women with tumor metastatic to lymph nodes, who have hormone receptor-positive tumors, are usually given adjuvant therapy with Tamoxifen rather than chemotherapy.

HAS INTERFERON BEEN DEMONSTRATED TO BE OF VALUE IN TREATING ADVANCED BREAST CANCER?

Interferon is the name for a family of medications that has a variety of complex actions. It can inhibit the growth of viruses as well as destroy tumor cells. It also has the ability to affect a person's immune system.

Unfortunately, although interferon initially appeared potentially promising as a therapeutic agent for recurrent, advanced breast cancer, several recent studies have failed to substantiate the results. Many studies are still under way, and it is possible that by using different types of interferon, different doses, other treatment schedules, or interferon in combination with other agents, improved efficacy may be demonstrated.

CHAPTER X

Breast Reconstruction Following Mastectomy

It is important for women who have been told that they have breast cancer and who are going to have a mastectomy to realize that breast reconstructive surgery may be available to them. This knowledge can vastly improve a woman's outlook and her ability to cope with the loss of her breast. On the eve of a mastectomy, it provides some comfort for a woman to know that, although she will be losing her breast, there is hope for her on many fronts—not only that her treatment will likely cure her tumor but also that, if she so desires, cosmetic surgery can subsequently be done to restore her silhouette.

Breast cancer surgery seems to precipitate a dual cause for concern. Besides being fearful because of the malignancy itself, patients are also worried about the cosmetic effects of the surgery. Knowing that reconstructive surgery can be done alleviates at least one concern. I suggest that a woman discuss breast reconstruction with her surgeon in the same conversation in which mastectomy is being explained.

The following example illustrates the remarkably positive effect that knowing about breast reconstructive surgery can have on a woman who is faced with the need for a mastectomy.

Carol Stone is a forty-six-year-old woman who was in the shower soaping herself when she felt a rock-hard mass in her breast, almost three inches long. She made an appointment to see her family doctor the next day, and was referred to a breast surgeon. As had been suspected the mass was found to be a breast cancer. Because of the size and the location of the tumor, the surgeon told Carol that it was inadvisable to treat it primarily with radiation, and that she would require a mastectomy.

Carol was depressed and afraid. Not only did she have to cope with the malignancy and the threat that it might be incurable, but she also had to deal with the immediate reality of the loss of her breast.

During the next week, she made appointments to see two other doctors, to get their opinions on whether she could be safely treated without having her breast removed. Both independently advised breast removal. But the second doctor had a lengthy discussion with Carol about the potential for breast reconstructive surgery, and this provided her with a new dimension of hope. By improving her outlook, it made her better able to cope with her forthcoming surgery.

The timing of the breast reconstructive surgery is itself rather controversial. This will depend partly upon the surgeon's philosophy, but also upon factors relating to the woman's tumor. If the tumor is noninvasive (premalignant) or quite small and localized, the breast surgeon is more inclined to consider that the reconstructive surgery can be done at the same time as the mastectomy. Some surgeons feel that, if the tumor is large, reconstruction should be delayed pending the pathologist's final evaluation of the local extent of the tumor and of possible spread of disease to the lymph nodes.

Some surgeons prefer to defer reconstructive surgery for six months or more, even when the prognostic features of the tumor are good (in other words, the tumor is small and there is no lymph node involvement), because they feel that waiting this long will improve the blood supply to the area, which will result in superior healing and therefore a better cosmetic effect. Others feel that this delay is unnecessary.

If the tumor is large or if several lymph nodes contain metastatic disease, some surgeons feel that there should be a delay of at least two years or even longer before reconstructive surgery. They consider that if a local recurrence is going to happen, there is a reasonable likelihood that it will do so in the first few years after the mastectomy, and placing the prosthesis should be delayed so that they can observe for such early recurrence before the surgical reconstruction is done. The presence of a breast prosthesis may theoretically interfere with the immediate diagnosis of early recurrent disease localized to the chest. Besides, it would be unfortunate to place a prosthesis prematurely, only to have to remove it so that a local recurrence could be treated.

On the other hand, some plastic surgeons feel that even women who have larger tumors can have reconstructive surgery right away without any adverse effect on their prognosis. Clearly, most women who desire breast reconstructive surgery would like to have it performed early on. However, the desire to "return to normal" as soon as possible must be balanced with what is thought to be safest for the woman, given the extent and biologic nature of her particular tumor. To determine what is appropriate, a woman must obtain advice from her own breast surgeon, perhaps with consultation from a plastic surgeon.

It is obviously important that the presence of an implant and breast reconstructive surgery not jeopardize the patient's chances of cure. If each woman is evaluated as an individual, and appropriate decisions are made based on her unique situation, postmastectomy breast reconstruction should not worsen the chances of cure. In fact, the availability of breast reconstructive surgery should actually decrease the overall mortality from breast cancer, since the knowledge that such surgery is available may prompt women with breast lumps to seek medical care as soon as they notice their lesions.

The best candidates for reconstructive surgery are patients whose tumors have been detected and treated early, another fact that should encourage women to participate in screening programs and to perform breast self-examination. However, once a reasonable amount of time has passed and the patient has remained free of recurrent disease, reconstructive surgery can also be performed on the woman who initially had a more advanced tumor.

Although there are records of breast reconstructive operations performed in the 1800s, it was not until the 1960s that the surgical procedure of breast implantation began to become more sophisticated. The availability of the silicone prosthesis has been a significant advance in breast reconstructive surgery, transforming it into a relatively simple and safe operation with an aesthetically pleasing outcome.

Breast reconstruction is performed by inserting under the skin and muscle a prosthesis matched as well as possible to the woman's other breast. One factor that has vastly enhanced the plastic surgeon's ability to perform easy and more aesthetic breast reconstructive surgery is the trend away from radical mastectomy in favor of the modified radical mastectomy, which, as we have seen, preserves the pectoralis muscle; it is under this muscle that the silicone prosthesis is placed.

The breast prosthesis usually does not drop from the forces of nature and age as a normal breast does. In addition, the size of a prosthesis that will be placed under the skin and muscle may not be as big as the woman's other breast if her breast is quite large. Therefore, if the woman's unaffected breast is extremely large or dropped, the plastic surgeon will usually recommend surgery on that breast to reduce its size or raise it to be symmetrical with the breast that was reconstructed following mastectomy. It is the plastic surgeon's goal not only to replace the breast that has been removed, but also to restore the woman's silhouette to a properly proportioned, balanced figure.

There are a few different ways in which a nipple can be made for the reconstructed breast. One approach is nipple banking, in which the nipple from the breast being removed is temporarily sewn on the thigh or abdomen and then is subsequently sewn back onto the new, reconstructed breast. Some doctors are concerned that if there are malignant cells in the nipple, nipple banking will allow them to be transplanted back onto the reconstructed breast. Another option, if a woman has large nipples, is to remove a portion of the nipple from her normal breast and share it with the reconstructed breast. This obviously gives an excellent color match, and is a good choice when appropriate. If the woman's normal nipple has a pink tint, tissue for the new nipple can be obtained from the posterior aricular sulcus (behind the ear). If the woman's normal nipple has a brown tint, tissue for the new nipple may be taken from the inner thigh. Occasionally, breast reconstruction is performed without making a nipple for the new breast, especially when the woman's prime concern is her appearance in clothing or a bathing suit. In many instances, however, women who undergo breast reconstructive surgery do have nipples made.

Reconstructive surgery can be performed on a woman who has had a radical mastectomy. However, the cosmetic results, while good, may be somewhat less satisfying than those achieved following the less extensive modified radical mastectomy. In addition, the operation that may be necessary to provide proper breast reconstruction following radical mastectomy is frequently more complex.

The operation that may be required is the latissimus dorsi myocutaneous flap reconstruction, more commonly referred to by patients as the back-flap operation. In this operation, the skin and latissimus dorsi muscle from the back are freed from part of their attachments and relocated anteriorly on the chest wall where the breast had been, in approximately the position of the removed pectoralis major muscle. The silicone prosthesis used to make the breast mound is then placed under the muscle.

This operation is obviously more extensive than the typical simple silicone implantation. Although the surgeon attempts, when possible, to take the latissimus dorsi muscle from a location that will not be apparent when the woman wears a bathing suit, the operation does require two incisions (in the area of the back muscle and in the area of the re-created breast) and therefore leaves two scars to heal. Hospitalization usually lasts longer than it does for the simpler reconstructive procedure following the modified radical mastectomy.

A new operation that has been used during the past few years is the rectus flap operation, in which muscle and skin from the abdomen are brought to the chest. This is a bigger operation, necessitating a longer hospital stay and probably carrying a greater potential for complications, but it may offer advantages for some women.

The optimal reconstructive procedure must be tailored to the individual needs of the patient. In arriving at a recommendation, the plastic surgeon will be guided by the nature of the previous treatment and his or her evaluation of the patient's remaining tissue.

The trend, which has evolved considerably over the past one or two decades, toward performing modified radical mastectomy rather than radical mastectomy, when the breast is to be removed, has probably encouraged women to have reconstructive surgery, given the simpler reconstructive operation and more attractive results if the woman's initial surgery was limited to the modified radical mastectomy. Still, the back flap procedure does offer an important option for reconstructive surgery for the woman who has very tight and limited chest wall skin, who has had such an extensive operation that she required a skin graft to cover her chest wall, who has had a radical mastectomy, or perhaps even for the woman who has had postmastectomy radiation therapy, which may impair the postreconstruction healing process.

There is another procedure that has several applications and may be particularly useful for the woman who has tight chest wall skin and does not want the back flap operation. In this operation, a tissue expander (a deflated mammary implant) is put in place under the chest wall skin. When it is originally implanted it is flat, but the deflated mammary implant has a valve under the skin, through which the breast prosthesis can be inflated with fluid. This is a bit like the valve on a beach ball, which we use to fill the ball with air. Each week, the physician inserts some fluid into the valve so that the prosthesis can be expanded.

Although this produces a tight sensation at first, the discomfort and tightness subside during the next several hours. This temporary breast expander prosthesis is expanded at weekly intervals until its size is satisfactory and the skin over the implant is adequately stretched; then the temporary prosthesis is replaced with a permanent prosthesis. Tissue expanders can be placed at the time of mastectomy, if the surgeon and the patient both feel that it is safe and appropriate to do so.

Breast reconstruction is simpler and more likely to be cosmetically satisfactory if the woman has had a modified radical mastectomy rather than a radical mastectomy. However, it is important for the woman who has a locally advanced tumor and whose surgeon recommends radical surgery to remember that if the surgeon does not do as extensive an initial surgical procedure as he or she feels is necessary, and the woman develops a local recurrence because of that, she will no longer have any opportunity for breast reconstructive surgery at all—and may have jeopardized her chances of cure as well.

During the past few years, many women who have early breast cancer have opted for a lumpectomy and radiation therapy rather than a mastectomy. It is quite possible that if this procedure is definitively proven to be equally effective in curing early breast cancer, and if women take proper care of their bodies so that any breast cancers that do develop are diagnosed when the lesions are still small, that reconstructive breast surgery may be less frequently necessary.

For patients who have been treated for breast cancer by lumpectomy and radiation therapy, the breast that previously harbored the cancer often ends up looking almost identical to the normal breast. This is usually not the case with breast reconstruction following mastectomy. Al-

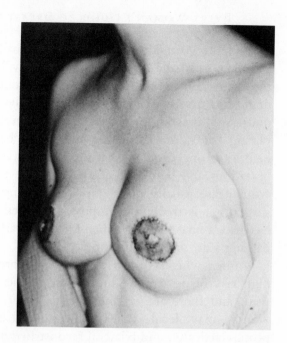

Figure 9

Figure 10

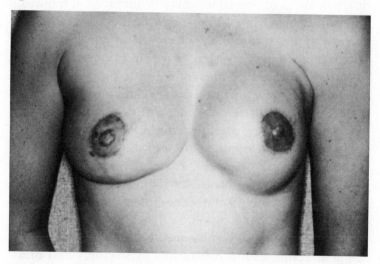

Figures 9–10 This patient was treated for breast cancer with a left modified radical mastectomy. The excellent cosmetic result was achieved with reconstructive surgery. (Photographs courtesy of Frederick N. Lukash, M.D.)

though the cosmetic result will occasionally be excellent and the normal and reconstructed breasts will look the same, the reconstructed breast will more commonly be easily distinguished from the normal breast when the woman is fully undressed. It is important for the woman who is contemplating breast reconstructive surgery to be aware of this before the operation, so that she won't have unrealistic expectations and be disappointed. Still, the results for most women are usually quite good. Following reconstructive surgery, it is frequently impossible to tell that a woman has had a mastectomy when she is wearing clothing, a bathing suit, or even just a bra.

Women who have had cancer in one breast are at very high risk of developing the disease in the other breast as well, and therefore, as mentioned earlier, occasionally a woman may decide to have the normal breast removed prophylactically, and bilateral reconstructive surgery. Two different types of procedures may be involved in removing a healthy breast from a high-risk woman. One is the subcutaneous mastectomy, in which the nipple-areola complex and external breast skin are left in place but the breast tissue underneath is removed; a breast prosthesis is then placed under the woman's own skin and nipple. Although the cosmetic result is excellent, and the chance of developing breast cancer greatly reduced, the woman still has some risk of developing breast cancer, since some of her own breast tissue is present. A simple mastectomy (complete removal of the breast, including the overlying skin and the nipple) should almost completely exclude the possibility of developing cancer in that breast. Breast reconstructive surgery can subsequently be performed. The cosmetic result with subcutaneous mastectomy and breast implant is better than with simple mastectomy and breast implant. However, if a woman is at such high risk and so fearful of developing breast cancer that she decides to have a normal breast removed, it seems more likely that she will also decide to have the surgery performed in the fashion that has the greatest likelihood of assuring the prevention of disease.

There are many variables that women must consider before deciding to have reconstructive surgery. One important factor is clearly what a woman's doctor tells her regarding her prognosis and the effects of the prosthesis. Some physicians feel that reconstructive surgery may make it more difficult to monitor for recurrent cancer. This becomes particularly significant for the woman who is statistically at high risk of developing a local recurrence, and it therefore must be discussed with the surgeon. All women who have had breast cancer, whether or not they have reconstructive surgery, must be carefully monitored afterward to watch for recurrent disease.

Obviously, a woman would not decide on reconstructive surgery if there were a serious possibility that it might jeopardize her chances of cure. There is some disagreement among doctors as to whether immediate reconstructive surgery can make it more difficult to diagnose recurrent breast cancer and whether this could in any way alter the outcome for a woman who was at high risk for developing a local recurrence.

Some women who have a mastectomy are at a time and stage in their lives when they are not very concerned about whether the breast is present, and are satisfied with wearing an external breast prosthesis. Many women do not want to undergo another hospitalization, surgical procedure, and anesthetic. In addition, the chance for good cosmetic results may not be very high for some women—those who require a skin graft, or who have had radiation therapy, extensive local disease, or a radical mastectomy—and it may require more than one operation to achieve a satisfactory result. Such women may also decide against attempting reconstruction.

Then, too, breast reconstructive surgery may represent a considerable expense for a woman and her family. Many insurance companies have to some extent come out of the dark ages and ceased to regard breast reconstructive surgery as "elective cosmetic surgery," for which the companies usually do not pay. Many more insurance companies now regard the procedure as indicated surgery, and are more likely to be willing to pay for it than they were a decade ago. I would advise a woman who is planning to undergo breast reconstructive surgery to find out her insurance company's reimbursement policies before she undergoes surgery, so that there are no unpleasant financial surprises. It is worthwhile to ascertain specifically whether and how much they are willing to reimburse, not only for the breast reconstruction itself, but also for the nipple reconstruction and for the operation in which the normal breast is altered to match the reconstructed breast. This is very important, since in some cases breast reconstructive surgery may consist of these three separate operations, which may be performed over the course of several months.

The decision to have breast reconstructive surgery does not have to be made immediately. Although most women who are interested in reconstruction request that it be done as soon as the surgeon feels it is appropriate, a woman may wait as long as a decade or more. While it is unusual to wait so long, I believe that it is psychologically very helpful for a woman to know she has this option.

Although I certainly do not advocate breast reconstructive surgery for every woman who has had a mastectomy, I think it is very important for a woman to understand that she has this available to her. If a woman knows that reconstruction can be performed after a mastectomy, she may be willing to seek medical help as soon as she finds a lump in her breast, particularly if she is aware that the earlier a tumor is found, the more likely she is to be able to undergo breast reconstructive surgery successfully. Besides, if on the eve of her mastectomy a woman realizes that reconstruction of the breast may be a reasonable possibility for her, this may help allay some of her anxieties.

Breast reconstructive surgery following a mastectomy may have a profoundly positive psychological impact. It may help a woman feel she is making a major step toward returning to a normal life. Many women who have chosen it feel that it has vastly improved their outlook and enhanced the quality of their lives.

CHAPTER XI

The Psychology of Breast Disease: Factors That Prevent Early Diagnosis

Women in the 1980s have become extremely conscious of their health and their bodies. They seem more inclined than ever before to exercise, to attend to their diets, and to be well informed about a variety of health-related issues. Yet it continues to amaze me that so many of these intelligent, sophisticated women are not performing monthly breast self-examination.

Of the women I see in the office for the first time, I would estimate that only twenty percent perform monthly breast self-examination. In speaking to my medical colleagues and reviewing the medical literature, I have found that this twenty-percent figure appears to be the average. Unfortunately, it seems that even when women have been instructed in breast self-examination, only about forty percent will continue to practice it on a regular basis. It is paradoxical that intelligent, well-informed, health-conscious women, who spend hours exercising and reading about health and nutrition, do not think it's important enough to perform an examination that is simple, painless, takes five minutes each month, and can help save their lives.

Their reasons are usually totally irrational: they are afraid, anxious, and don't believe it can happen to them. But with a risk of one in eleven, this is much too great a gamble.

All the avoidance, denial, and anxiety in the world will not prevent a woman from developing breast cancer, but these factors do keep women from examining their breasts. It must be stressed over and over again that just by virtue of being women, we are all at great risk of developing breast cancer. For some groups of women the risk is considerably greater, for others somewhat less, but even the theoretically "low-risk" woman remains at considerable risk.

Whether a woman does or does not examine her breasts, she still has the same likelihood of developing breast cancer. However, if she faithfully performs monthly breast self-examination, it is probable that any malignancy she does develop will be found early enough for her to be cured. In addition, she gives herself a greater chance of being able to preserve her breast and be cured primarily with radiation therapy, or, if she chooses mastectomy, to have less radical surgery and be a better candidate for breast reconstruction.

For some women, anxiety results in paralysis and inaction. Other women are able to harness the anxiety and make absolutely certain that they perform monthly breast self-examination. So many women are well informed, know the risks of breast cancer, have been instructed in breast self-examination, know what they should do and why— and yet do nothing. The psychological reasons behind this illogical inactivity include denial, anxiety, repression, narcissism, indecision, and fear.

If psychological reasons prevent women from examining themselves, perhaps psychology can be mobilized to encourage women to perform breast self-examination; perhaps group psychology should be used. For many different types of problems that we have, we use the support of a group to motivate ourselves. People who have difficulty dieting may join Weight Watchers; those who wish to stop smoking may participate in Smokenders or some other group; people who want to exercise but are not independently motivated may perform better if they join an exercise class. Support groups have flourished so that we can help one another in achieving common goals. There are groups for single parents, for parents with chronically ill children, etc.

The energy of a group is very powerful, and it can motivate people and convert their energy and concern into activity. Since breast cancer is one of the most common serious medical problems that women may develop, and since the purpose of women's groups is for women to work together to help one another, perhaps what we should be doing at the end of each meeting of a group of women, whether it's a meeting of NOW, a women's professional organization, a mothers' group, or a local card group, is talking for a few minutes about one of the most serious threats to our well-being, and agreeing to take steps to reduce our risk of dying of breast cancer. If you sit in a room with other women, whether there are six, sixty, or six hundred, there is a high probability that one or many of you will develop breast cancer. We use our groups to help us with so many issues, from professional networking to emotional support. Shouldn't we use them to help save lives? If after every meeting of a group of women most of the members went home determined to perform monthly breast self-examination, this alone would probably reduce the annual mortality from breast cancer.

When I thought about this idea, it first seemed to me to be simplistic and perhaps a bit naïve. But, the more I consider it, what truly seemed naïve and ridiculous was that we have a way to prevent death and pain on a large scale that takes only five minutes a month and requires no special skills or equipment—and almost eighty percent of women do nothing about it.

The underlying psychological principle behind any support group is indeed simplistic and basic: people who have a particular interest or need may be better able to harness their energies and tackle their problems with the support of a group of people who share that interest or need. Motivating people to take appropriate care of their bodies seems to be a perfect issue for a support group to tackle. If it seems silly to anyone for women to use a group to encourage one another to be examining our own breasts, perhaps this relates to feelings about our breasts, childish notions that are remnants of our adolescent fantasies and taboos, rather than to what is clearly good common sense about maintaining our health.

Personally, I would find it much more positive to see our women's support groups reminding us and encouraging us to perform self-examination than to have the need for more support groups for increasing numbers of women who have recurrent breast cancer. Support groups for women with advanced cancer can obviously be extremely useful, but if we put enough emphasis on prevention and early detection, perhaps we can reduce the numbers of women who have advanced disease.

Sharon Bromley Christianson had worked as a banker since she graduated from business school fifteen years earlier. Three years ago, when she was thirty-six, Sharon and her husband, Bob, decided to have a child. When Jessica was born, Sharon wanted to spend some time at home with the baby. She immersed herself in activities with her newborn, which she enjoyed tremendously. Putting her organizational talents to work, Sharon created a mothers-and-toddlers group for her neighborhood. Two afternoons a week, fifteen mothers and their young children would gather. Although most of the mothers' attention was directed toward supervising and playing with the children, there was always a good deal of helpful conversation among them. The range of topics was broad, and always practical—how to get the children to go to sleep, how to find a good babysitter, at what age the children should start nursery school and which local school was the best, how to keep husbands appropriately involved with the childrens' development, etc. During the course of the first several months, dozens of issues arose, and several members of the group usually had practical and helpful advice as to how they had approached the problems. As the women got to know one another well, they began to rely on each other more and more for support.

During the first few weeks of March, Pat Roberts had some family problems but asked if she could drop off her son Eric at the play-group sessions so that he could be with his friends even though she couldn't stay. In late March, when Pat returned to the group, she explained to her friends that her absence had been due to her mother's need for help during and after her surgery for breast cancer. The women expressed their concern for Pat's mother and asked how she was coming along. Pat was very upset: her mother's cancer wasn't diagnosed until it was quite large and the tumor had already spread to several lymph nodes. This precipitated a lengthy discussion about the early diagnosis of breast cancer and the importance of performing breast self-examination. By the end of the afternoon, all of the women realized that breast cancer represented a significant threat to them, and therefore to their families. They had responsibilities to themselves and to their children. Each woman left, committed to the intention of performing breast self-examination.

During the ensuing weeks, there was no talk about breast disease. Summer was approaching. Conversations were about gardens, vacations, and visits by in-laws.

As time passed, Pat was of course still helping her mother to recuperate, and the problem of breast cancer was certainly in her thoughts. In early June, she reminded her friends of their earlier conversations about breast self-examination. Of the fifteen women in the group, ten had followed through and performed it. Two-thirds wasn't too bad, she thought. However, they reminded one another that it needed to be done monthly. And they urged their five friends not to be delinquent.

At their next meeting, Sharon was quite upset. She told her friends that she had finally performed breast self-examination, and had discovered a lump. She saw her doctor that day. Although the doctor felt that the mass was probably benign, she had advised Sharon to see a surgeon, and told her that she would likely require a biopsy. The following week Sharon had the biopsy. To everyone's relief, the mass was benign. However, Sharon kept on doing monthly breast self-examination. Her friends in the mothers-and-toddlers group continued to remind one another about it. They also spoke about it with other friends outside the group.

Although for some women the thought of performing breast self-examination generates considerable anxiety, this pales by comparison to the anxiety generated in almost all women should they find a lump in their breasts. In an instant, dozens of thoughts flash through such a woman's mind. Is it malignant? Will I lose my breast? Will I die? Will I suffer? What will happen to my family, my career?

Whether the woman's breast abnormality is ultimately determined to be benign or malignant, the interval between first discovering a lump, finally having a biopsy, and hearing whether the lesion is benign or malignant can be devastating. The time frame for this may be as long as a month, occasionally longer. For some people, the uncertainty triggers an even greater emotional reaction than the reality. It is often easier to cope with facts, even unpleasant ones, than to be suspended in a state of uncertainty.

I have seen a few psychologically healthy types of approaches that women have had once they have found a lump, and a few seriously pathologic reactions. Obviously, once a woman finds a mass in her breast, the only appropriate action is to make an appointment with a doctor. In addition, depending upon the individual's psychological makeup, she may do a variety of things. She may read extensively about breast disease, she may discuss the situation with friends and family, she may call the American Cancer Society, she may decide to get more than one opinion, or she may decide to put the lump completely out of her mind until she sees a physician. Any coping mechanisms that a woman chooses, and any steps she takes to inform herself about breast disease and to help herself physically and psychologically, are almost always in her best medical and emotional interest.

Unfortunately, some people use "coping mechanisms" that employ illogical reasoning and are ultimately detrimental to their physical and emotional well-being. I have seen women with enormous tumors who did not seek medical attention for months or years because they were pretending that if they ignored their tumors they problem would disappear, or because they "didn't want to start something." The tumors themselves are what "start something," and it's just common sense that getting prompt and appropriate medical care is the best way to prevent a serious situation from further deteriorating.

Yet there are people who feel malignancies when they are small, watch them as they grow, deny that they are harmful or even present, and wait until the situation ultimately becomes acute and incurable before seeking care. A few patients like this come to me each year with various types of malignancies, and it is dreadful to see women who could have been cured had they sought medical attention when they first discovered the problem, lose that opportunity because of illogical and irrational thinking. Perhaps if physicians, the media, and support groups continue to emphasize to women that breast cancer detected early is usually curable, and that early disease can frequently be cured with excellent cosmetic results, we will see less of this frightening, irrational behavior.

Some amount of denial can be good. For instance, a woman who finds a breast mass, makes an appointment to see her physician, and then decides to put the mass out of her thoughts until the doctor tells her what it is, is using denial in a healthy way. This woman has arranged for proper and prompt medical attention, but has also decided not to worry about the mass. For some people, denial can help to allay the immense anxiety that people often experience in the interval of time between finding a lump and learning whether it is benign or malignant. But whereas denial and repression can be important psychological tools for coping, they become dangerous when they are employed pathologically, keeping a person from seeking appropriate medical attention for a potentially serious problem. Severe stress may result in a pattern of illogical reasoning and inappropriate behavior. People may not seek medical care because they are afraid of suffering, yet by not receiving appropriate and timely medical care they are actually making it more likely that they will suffer.

In 1973 a poll was conducted to evaluate women's fears regarding breast cancer, to determine which possibility women feared more, having a malignancy or losing a breast. Fifty-nine percent of the women said they were more afraid of the malignancy, but twenty-three percent indicated that they were more concerned about losing a breast. Women have clearly become more liberated, and I assume that the results would be somewhat different in this decade. However, the most important point to stress once again is that if breast tumors are diagnosed early enough, women may be able to be cured and to save their breasts. By facing fears head-on, examining themselves, and seeking immediate medical attention for any abnormality that is discovered, women can conquer both very real fears.

It is obviously not easy, and I certainly don't mean to indicate that it is anything other than emotionally traumatic for almost any woman, regardless of her age and personal circumstances, to find a mass in her breast. Almost every woman in such a situation will experience anxiety, fear, stress, depression, hostility, and a vast array of other emotions. These will be common reactions to a very harrowing and stressful situation. However, it is essential that a woman use all her emotional resources and fortitude to insure that she receives prompt and proper medical care. It's normal to cry, to be hostile, to be anxious—people respond to traumatic circumstances in such a wide variety of ways. But, whatever the psychological response, it must not interfere with a woman's receiving prompt medical care.

CHAPTER XII

Psychological Adaptation of the Breast-Cancer Patient

"Once I learned that the lump was malignant, I felt hostility toward all other healthy women. I was angry that it had happened to me and wished that it had happened instead to one of them."

"When the doctor told me that he had palpated a mass in my breast which he was certain was a malignancy, I denied that this could be possible. I became angry at him and, despite repeated urging, I refused to even have a biopsy for several weeks."

"When the doctor told me that I had breast cancer, I bought several books about it and spoke to everyone I could find who knew anything about the disease. Having as much information as possible helped me to be in control."

"My major concern, when I learned that I had breast cancer, was what would happen to my children if I was unable to care for them."

Almost all people find it devastating to learn they have a malignancy. A vast range of thoughts and emotions run through people's minds in a split second as they realize the implications of their illness. They may feel angry, depressed, anxious, fearful, or even optimistic. They may worry about their lives, their families, the pain that may lie in store for them, and how the quality of their lives will change. When a woman is told she has breast cancer, she faces a crisis of perhaps the greatest magnitude that she has ever had to face. There is no correct way to react, but the ultimate goal must be the restoration of good psychological as well as physical health.

As children grow up, they develop certain behavior patterns that usually remain with them throughout their adult lives. Therefore, an adult's response to a crisis situation is in part predetermined by previous life experiences and the way former traumas were approached. So, to some extent, a woman's way of dealing with learning that she has breast cancer may be predictable. A person who feels most comfortable being in control may want to learn as much about the disease as possible, know all the facts, and work closely with the doctor in determining her therapy. A person who typically copes with problems by denying their existence may not want to hear any details of her illness and may want her family or doctor to make all the decisions and provide her with sketchy information only. A vast spectrum of behavior and response may be exhibited by a woman who has breast cancer. The woman needs to work through her reactions of anger, fear, depression, denial, or whatever she is experiencing, so that she can eventually reach a reasonably comfortable acceptance and equilibrium. Unfortunately, a woman frequently suffers a good deal of psychological pain before reaching such a relatively stable emotional position. Many women find the trauma of the breast cancer and its aftermath remaining in their minds for years, perhaps forever. It may take an enormous amount of external support and inner fortitude to conquer the psychological trauma.

Many women, upon being told they have breast cancer, are angry, and expressing this hostility is usually helpful. They are angry at their fate—that it happened to them and not someone else. They want to know why all those other women were spared and why they themselves were afflicted. They may want to scream and cry, and they probably should. In any case, they must realize that it's okay to be angry or fearful—that, whatever their feelings are, they can be expressed.

Most people in this type of situation must let out their anger and their fear as a first step in dealing with the crisis. Some choose to repress their anger and act stoically as a coping mechanism, and this may help them get through the experience, but repression may not be healthy. If people act stoically because they believe it is what is expected of them, meanwhile not expressing or working through the anger they truly feel, they may actually delay their ultimate psychological recovery. In a situation like this, where such extreme anger may be evoked, it is probably better to express it than deny it.

There is one caveat, though. Often the anger a cancer patient feels is so overwhelming and so diffuse that she keeps lashing out at her family and friends. They may start out sympathetic, but eventually, if the hostile behavior is too intense and persistent, it may damage the woman's relationship with her family and friends and make her feel even more isolated in her pain. Patients also occasionally express inappropriate anger at the doctors and nurses who are providing care for them. Health-care providers have been trained to understand this behavior and can usually deal with it effectively, but if it is extreme, this type of behavior can impair the doctor-patient relationship.

Beatrice Fromm had always been considered "the strong one" by her family and friends. She was the oldest of three sisters, and ever since she was seventeen, when her mother died of breast cancer, her two younger sisters had looked to her as a source of guidance and help.

Beatrice became a doctor, specializing in heart disease. She married an obstetrician and they had two lovely children. Because of her husband's long and unpredictable work schedule, Beatrice bore most of the responsibility for organizing the household and raising the children.

When her two daughters were in their teens, Beatrice developed breast cancer. Since she had obviously been aware of her risk for developing the disease, she had been performing monthly breast self-examination, and was fortunate enough to discover the malignancy when it was only the size of a small pea, with all the lymph nodes still free of tumor. Beatrice was able to be treated with a lumpectomy, removal of lymph nodes in the underarm, and radiation therapy.

Beatrice knew that she was in some ways fortunate to have discovered the tumor when it was so small; her prognosis was excellent and she had a very good cosmetic result as well. Still, she was angry and afraid—angry that she had been at high risk because of her mother's illness, angry at her mother for dying and leaving her, and angry that she had breast cancer rather than someone else. She was also worried, afraid of developing recurrent cancer and dying of the disease, afraid of leaving her children without a mother, and afraid that one day her daughters might also develop cancer.

Beatrice was not the type to express her fears and anxieties to others. After all, she was "the strong one." She had had to handle her problems as a teen-ager, and now she had to handle her own problems and those of others, too, as a doctor, a mother, and a wife.

Just as Beatrice had done with all the problems in her life, she kept her fears and anger to herself. Nevertheless, her hostility became more and more apparent to those around her. She was short-tempered at work, and her patients began to notice the absence of the warmth and empathy they had previously felt from her. At home, she had no patience for her children's usual teen-age problems.

Besides being angry and afraid, Beatrice was unwilling to accept the emotional support that so many of her family and friends were trying to give her. She abruptly cut off her husband whenever he tried to be encouraging or helpful.

Thus, during the few months following her illness, Beatrice had not just shut her family out and refused their support and help, but had truly become hostile to them.

Beatrice's husband felt she was obviously on a destructive course: though she was probably cured physically of her disease, she was developing serious emotional problems. So he spoke with Beatrice's physician about her psychological inability to respond to help, to verbalize her fears and anger, and to cope. They decided that Beatrice urgently needed psychological counseling, and they convinced her to have it. With this help, her outlook and her ability to cope have vastly improved. Beatrice realized that she would have been better off discussing her angers and fears with the people she loved. She had tried to hide and repress them. However, the negative feelings were so strong that they just manifested themselves in other ways.

Depression is another emotion people frequently experience when they learn they have a malignancy. This may occur in a person who is not typically depressed, and it is somewhat different from chronic depression in that it is a response to a life crisis. As is the case with anger, it is probably better to acknowledge your feelings of depression. Don't be afraid to cry.

Women with malignancies often experience fear as well. Much of it involves very real and important issues with which the woman must cope. She may be worried about how her family could manage without her, particularly if she is the mother of young children, if she is responsible for the care of elderly parents or an ailing spouse, or if the family is dependent on her income. She may fear the possibility of losing a breast, of suffering physically or psychologically, or of dying. She may fear losing the love of her spouse or her friends, or the inability to become involved in new relationships. She may be concerned about the effects of the malignancy on her career and her professional life.

Many of these fears are very real concerns. They are issues that the patient eventually identifies and copes with as best she can. The particular fears that a woman has will depend upon her priorities and the circumstances of her life. Some of them have no simple solutions. Occasionally, however, the fear is worse than the reality. The terrifying scenarios that the patient imagines may be much worse than what the future holds in store—but the psychological pain is real. It is not uncommon for women to experience sleep disorders and nightmares, sometimes for prolonged periods.

One reaction to breast cancer that is fortunately uncommon is that of guilt. Some people believe that they have been afflicted as a punishment for improper thoughts or actions, particularly in relation to sexual behavior. Women also may feel guilty and fearful that they will no longer be "sexually complete" for their partners.

Many people deal with malignancy by using some amount of denial (ignoring the facts), and, as mentioned earlier, to the extent that it helps them cope, it may be helpful. Very few people can comfortably consider the mortality statistics for women with breast cancer and accept the possibility that they themselves might become a negative statistic. It can be painful to live with thoughts of potential death or suffering. Some amount of denial may help a woman maintain a positive approach to her situation and help her enjoy her life. Denial that makes it easier to cope with life events is, after all, used to some extent by most people in their day-to-day activities. Yet, although some denial can be helpful, there are occasional instances in which I have seen it carried to extremes, to the real detriment of the cancer patient. I have seen women refuse required therapy, deny to themselves that they had a malignancy at all, ignore their follow-up appointments, and deny the presence of recurrent cancer. When denial prevents someone from seeking required treatment, it may be life-threatening, no longer a survival mechanism at all.

Particularly in recent years, I find that increasing numbers of women cope best by learning the facts and feeling that they are in control of the situation. They feel that by being fully informed they can help control their own destiny. They read about the illness, ask friends who have had similar problems, and frequently seek a second opinion regarding their illness and possible methods of treatment. An ever-diminishing number of patients find the facts so anxiety-provoking that they prefer to be told by their doctor or family what course they should take, with a minimum amount of detail. For many patients, the uncertainty is what produces the greatest anxiety, and once they have information and feel more in control of their lives, they are better able to cope.

Unfortunately, the emotional suffering that a woman who has been diagnosed as having breast cancer will experience persists for unpredictable lengths of time. Though the acute pain may be brief, many women go on feeling the anger and fear for several years. Still, most people do confront the problem head-on. They realize that, despite their severe emotional distress, they must be able to resolve their conflicts and look toward the future. This is not to imply that their psychological pain immediately vanishes, but it will diminish as they look forward to and resume the activities and interests that they were involved with before becoming ill.

A woman usually discovers she has breast cancer very suddenly. A previously completely healthy woman, often in the prime of her life, may be feeling fine one minute and acquire this devastating information the next. She therefore has no time to prepare herself psychologically.

Eventually, as I've already indicated, most breast-cancer patients do confront and cope with their illness. Fortunately, they almost never have to do this completely alone. They can draw on the strength of their family and friends, support groups, doctors, social workers, and therapists. Even though the ultimate emotional resolution must occur from within, these individuals can help ease the transition.

The sensitive physician can be an enormous source of emotional strength and guidance. Most doctors who care for large numbers of patients with malignancies aim not only to cure the physical illness but to alleviate the psychological traumas as well. This means attempting to understand the patient as an individual, since the psychological needs of different patients vary considerably. Not every doctor will have the resources and training to deal appropriately with the emotional needs of every patient. Doctors will, therefore, often enlist the support of other members of the health-care team. Enormous psychological assistance and guidance can be provided by properly trained and motivated nurses and social workers. However, most physicians who care for women with malignancies are attuned to the immense psychological trauma that the illness creates and attempt to approach each patient in terms reflecting her psychological as well as physical needs.

Since breast cancer is so common, most women also have access to breast-cancer support groups, often starting while they are still patients in the hospital. These groups can be a great source of strength. It is important for women to realize how many others are confronting a similar problem and to know how many have successfully dealt with it. The groups may provide an excellent outlet for an immediate release of anger, pain, and fear, as well as an opportunity for an exchange of questions, advice, and practical information.

The Reach to Recovery program of the American Cancer Society may offer invaluable practical and psychological assistance to the woman with breast cancer. Once her doctor has indicated that a patient is ready, a Reach to Recovery volunteer can visit her. The volunteer is a woman who has been treated for breast cancer, has recovered, and has been trained to help the new patient. It is of tremendous value for the patient who has just developed breast cancer to see another woman who has confronted the same problem and made a successful recovery, both physical and emotional. Of course, the Reach to Recovery program is likely to be of great psychological benefit for the volunteer as well: it should be an enormous source of pride for the volunteer to realize that she has been able to conquer the trauma of her own illness and to help someone else cope.

Family and friends are often a source of great strength and may assist considerably in a woman's psychological recovery. Under optimal circumstances, they may be the woman's ideal support group. They are with her most, understand her best, and may be uniquely well equipped to help her.

Of course, they are people, too, with their own needs and problems, and occasionally the dynamics of the relationships are such that family and friends (even sincere, well-meaning ones) may do things that harm rather than assist the woman's psychological recovery. Their own fears of the possibility of losing a loved one may cause them to transmit a sense of gloom and depression to the patient. Alternatively, they may try so hard to create an aura of optimism that they give the patient unrealistic expectations, which may be dangerous if it prevents her from seeking or accepting proper medical care. Also, it may ultimately destroy the woman's trust in her family and her doctor, since their assurances have proven unwarranted.

Occasionally, family and friends may take an approach that is wrong for the woman's immediate needs. She may still be at the stage when what she needs is sympathy, while her friends and relatives are admonishing her to pull herself together. Alternatively, she may have reached the point where she is ready to draw upon all her inner fortitude and courage and reintegrate her life, while her relatives and friends are continuing to try to protect her from the situation and shield her from having to deal with the truth.

Besides these difficulties in relationships with friends and relatives who truly do mean well, there are often situations in which a woman had significant difficulties in the dynamics of her family relationships that predated the breast cancer. She may have had a poor or even a hostile relationship with her spouse or her children. Particularly if her relationship with her spouse has been tenuous, she may fear that he will not stand by her.

Occasionally, people would prefer to discuss their illness with a total stranger; they may even speak of the malignancy in great detail with a person whom they happen to be seated next to on a plane, though they refrain from having such an intimate conversation about the disease with their family. These people often fear that their loved ones will reject them, that the illness will stress their family relationships past what those relationships can handle. They are so concerned about being rejected by their family that they prefer to enlist the support of strangers, or to deal with their problems alone. Though this assessment of the family's reaction may be correct, it is frequently completely unwarranted, based on the woman's insecurities rather than on how people really feel about her.

Occasionally, the illness may even draw the family together. The fear of losing a loved one often jolts a family with the realization of just how much they do love her and how important she is to them. I have seen several spouses who had previously been wandering and thoughtless and who in times of illness and crisis became strong supports, pillars of loving strength for their wives, standing by them and helping them through the illness and thereafter.

Some patients with a malignancy can be helped considerably by enlisting the support of a psychiatrist. Although it is a less common reaction now than it used to be, there are still people who feel that there is some stigma attached to needing psychiatric care. It must be repeatedly emphasized that the role of a psychiatrist is not necessarily to care for people who are "crazy." Cancer provokes a serious life crisis, and psychiatrists and therapists can help a patient and her family to cope with it. Even when a woman has a loving, caring family, they may be unable to support her emotionally because her illness has precipitated a life crisis for them as well. Mental-health professionals can help the woman and may also work with the family. Psychiatrists may feel that certain women who have cancer would also benefit from antidepressant medication.

The support that a religious leader may offer should not be overlooked. Women who have a strong religious affiliation may think immediately of this as a source of assistance. However, even those who have not maintained strong religious ties may find that their religious leader is well equipped to help them and can be a source of sage advice as well as comfort through this period of crisis.

For some women, physical recovery from malignancy may be easier to achieve than psychological recovery. Long after the cancer has been cured, emotional scars may persist. Fortunately, health-care professionals seem to be increasingly attuned to this and continue to make inroads in easing the psychological stresses of the disease. Though it may take years for a woman to reattain her former level of emotional equilibrium, and unfortunately some women are never able to achieve this, the goal for which the patient, her family, and her doctor all strive is the combination of physical and emotional well-being. It is not enough to conquer the cancer; the emotional effects of the illness must be treated as well.

CHAPTER XIII

Sexual Readjustment Following Mastectomy

Sexual readjustment following breast-cancer surgery is frequently a mirror that reflects several other aspects of the woman's psychological response to her illness, one good indicator of how well she has come to terms with her disease. At the same time, comfortable sexual adjustment often acts to help a woman regain her self-esteem as well.

The two features about the development of breast cancer that appear to be most traumatic to a woman, as discussed earlier, are the fear of mortality and the fear of losing the breast. Concerns relating to the loss of the breast are often grounded in a woman's worries about altered body image and attractiveness. If she resumes an emotionally satisfying sexual relationship, these concerns usually diminish. The woman can understand and realize that, despite her physical alteration, she is the same person, who can love and be loved.

The breast-cancer patient's sexual involvement with her partner when she returns home after surgery will depend in large measure upon what this relationship was like before she went to the hospital. It will depend upon the emotional makeup of the individuals involved and upon the dynamics of their relationship as it has existed over time.

There are so many possibilities here. Breast cancer is egalitarian: although some women are at greater risk than others of developing the disease, all women are potentially at risk. They may be happily married, unhappily married, single, divorced, separated, or widowed. They may have been sexually active and be concerned about their future sexuality, or they may have little interest in sex.

For any woman who has had a mastectomy (for any woman at all, for that matter), the goal is to arrive at a degree of sexual adjustment that is pleasing and appropriate for her. The goal of cancer treatment is to rehabilitate the patient physically and emotionally, as I have said, so that she is not just alive but happy to be alive and enjoying life. If a breast cancer patient has been cured of her tumor but is permanently distraught and never psychologically rehabilitated, then only part of the therapy has been attended to. And since sexuality is, for many women, a significant part of life, it is important that women be well aware that having a mastectomy does not signify the end of sexual relationships.

Although circumstances will vary from woman to woman, let us first consider the most common situation: a woman who has had a reasonably good emotional and sexual relationship with her husband and who now returns home following a mastectomy.

A multitude of factors will contribute to whether the patient achieves a satisfactory sexual readjustment. One relates to how well the woman herself copes with having lost her breast. Many women are somewhat depressed following a mastectomy, and depression from any source usually results in a vastly diminished sex drive.

Clearly, another factor in the woman's sexual adjustment following her mastectomy will be her husband's ability to cope with her cancer and with the loss of her breast.

A woman who has recently been confronted with breast cancer and mastectomy may well find it infuriating that she must consider not only her own emotions and stress at this time, but also her husband's difficulties in coping. The fact is, however, that at this time the husband is usually quite fearful about losing his wife and about potential changes in their relationship; the breast cancer commonly precipitates emotional trauma for him as well.

The sexual difficulties some couples encounter following mastectomy are to an extent the result of a self-fulfilling prophecy. Each spouse is a little cautious, uncertain about the feelings and desires of the other, and is usually afraid to discuss things openly, for fear of causing more emotional distress. The husband may be afraid to approach his wife sexually. He may be afraid to hurt her, fearful that she is too weak, or concerned that she is not emotionally ready. Following a mastectomy, almost all women worry about their sexual desirability; a woman will often take the fact that her husband has not initiated sex as a confirmation of her fears that she is no longer desirable. Feeling rejected, and questioning her own desirability, the wife may be afraid to initiate sex, for fear of experiencing further rejection and confirmation of her self-doubts.

The longer this situation persists, the more vicious a cycle it becomes. It helps if sexual relations resume early on, as soon as there is physical and emotional readiness to do so.

Among the many reasons why the breast-cancer patient and her spouse should communicate effectively and openly, it will certainly tend to improve their sexual relationship. During this time, when misunderstanding and confusion by both partners are not uncommon, it is important to know you can express your feelings to your partner. Many husbands and wives are uncomfortable about discussing their sexual feelings and needs; it usually becomes even more difficult to do so following a mastectomy. Though you may be afraid to bring your feelings out into the open, *not* discussing them may well cause problems to fester.

In addition to discussing their emotional needs and their readiness to resume sexual relations, couples must understand some specific medical considerations. A woman recovering from a mastectomy may have trouble supporting herself with her arm on the side of the operation, and it is extremely important for her to make sure the arm sustains no trauma. Her chest may be uncomfortably sensitive to pressure or may be numb, and special care must be taken if this is the case.

A woman's physical and emotional relationship with her husband after her mastectomy depends a lot on what the relationship was like before the mastectomy. If the marriage was rocky and interaction was tenuous at all levels, the relationship may not be able to withstand this additional crisis. On the other hand, many women who are treated for breast cancer report that their husbands surprise them with a degree of tenderness and affection that they had not exhibited for several decades. For many couples for whom the years of familiarity had caused a drifting apart, the crisis of serious illness results in a combining of resources and strengths and a new closeness in the relationship.

Some women are not interested in sexual readjustment after mastectomy. There is nothing inherently wrong with this attitude, providing that other factors are considered. Is this lack of interest in sexual rehabilitation an indication that the woman feels a sense of hopelessness about her disease? Is the woman having emotional difficulties in readjusting to other aspects of life? Has her relationship with her husband returned to a mutually supportive and emotionally satisfying one, despite the absence of sexual interaction?

A healthy readjustment following breast-cancer surgery does not necessarily imply a return to sexual activity. However, most women do feel that their sexuality is a pleasant part of their lives, and a positive component of their relationship with their partners.

It is obviously perfectly acceptable for a woman to decide that she is not interested in a physical relationship, whether or not she has had breast cancer. On the other hand, it is unfortunate for a woman who has previously had a satisfying sex life to give up that part of her life out of fear (almost always unwarranted) that she will be rejected by her partner because she has lost her breast.

Following the wife's developing breast cancer, husbands occasionally have their own sexual problems, including difficulty having or maintaining an erection. This often relates to the enormous stress that the cancer provokes, in the individuals and in the relationship. The first step in approaching this difficulty is to maintain a warm, caring, close relationship. Whether or not the couple is having intercourse, they should be tender with each other, and kiss and caress. The husband's difficulties most often represent an acute response to this stressful situation and are likely to be of brief duration. Good communication between the partners and an affectionate relationship will frequently help alleviate the problem. If it persists, short-term sexual counseling is usually quite effective.

These issues involving sexual readjustment following mastectomy involve common reactions to very stressful circumstances, and can be addressed and overcome. Certain other responses to breast cancer and mastectomy, however, are more dangerous to the woman's emotional well-being, occasionally to the point of being pathological. As mentioned earlier, some women have indicated that they are convinced they have developed breast cancer as punishment for previous sexual activity. The weight of such guilt is enormous, and frequently impairs the woman's psychological recovery in general, as well as her ability to resume normal sexual relations.

Another fear a woman occasionally harbors that is not only incorrect but also harmful is that if her other breast is ever stimulated, it, too, will become diseased. Occasionally, a woman's spouse will withdraw from her and be afraid to resume sexual relations because he is concerned that the malignancy may be transmitted to him, or, if his wife has received radiation therapy, that she may be radioactive. These fears, which have no known medical validity, would obviously be damaging to any relationship.

Sometimes a woman is so relieved to be cured of her cancer that she feels she may be asking for too much to expect an enjoyable sex life as well. In helping patients who have had a malignancy, I have found that such an attitude toward the disease can be harmful. I always encourage my patients to try to resume their lives in a positive way. It seems so unfortunate for a woman to go through all the physical and emotional strains that she does in her attempt to be cured of her cancer if she is not going to have the most complete and enjoyable life that she can afterward.

A few women who have had breast cancer and a mastectomy will attempt to increase their sexual activity dramatically, seeking out multiple partners to prove to themselves that they are still desirable. This type of behavior is usually detrimental to the woman. She will probably end up feeling a loss of self-esteem, rather than the hoped-for increase in confidence.

Some patients who have been treated for breast cancer may do well with some short-term sexual or psychological counseling. Patients are frequently reluctant to discuss sexual problems with their surgeons, although many doctors have had extensive experience with breast-cancer patients and will be able to offer assistance with these problems. If the surgeon does not feel able to provide a patient with sexual counseling and the patient feels it would be useful, she and her partner might benefit from outside professional sexual counseling. Expressing their fears and anxieties to a professional is occasionally all they need to improve their relationship dramatically. Short-term sexual counseling is frequently helpful in getting the two partners to open up to each other; once they are able to express the flood of emotions and thoughts they have been keeping dammed up, they often find their sexual feelings and sex life return to normal.

One question I am frequently asked is whether a woman should reveal her mastectomy scar to her partner, and particularly whether she should fully undress for intercourse. The only way I can appropriately answer this question is to relate the sentiments of some of the breast-cancer patients I have spoken to.

Some women feel that, to readjust properly both emotionally and sexually, they must get used to their scars and accept them, and that they must encourage their partners to accept these scars as part of reality as well. They feel that only then can they get over their trauma and carry on with their lives in the most positive fashion. Others, however, feel that, although they have come to terms with their illness, there is no reason to force themselves and their partners to be repeatedly reminded of it. Some women never show their husbands their scars. Women should do what is most comfortable, physically and emotionally, for both themselves and their partners.

Many women choose to wear their breast prostheses (some are lightweight and specifically designed to be comfortable to sleep in) while having sexual relations. Opinions are divided among patients who have had a mastectomy as to whether it is psychologically helpful to do so. I think that if it helps either the woman or her partner psychologically or physically to have her wear the prosthesis during sexual relations, she should by all means do so. Occasionally, women have complained that it is physically uncomfortable to wear the breast prosthesis while they are having sex, and that it puts pressure on the chest. Again, each woman must decide what is appropriate for her own needs.

In summary, it is obvious that learning she has breast cancer and undergoing a mastectomy will have a profound psychological impact on a woman. The feelings of anxiety, depression, and fear that occur almost always result in at least a transient decline in any interest in sexuality. The woman's sexual activity is also significantly affected by all the concerns of her partner. He is often puzzled and worried, and does not know what his wife wants. Is she feeling well enough, physically and emotionally, to engage in sexual activity? How will she interpret his advances and desires? How will he react to his wife's body? The husband is often so confused by the vast and conflicting range of his own emotions, and his fears and concerns for his wife, that he becomes paralyzed and does not initiate any sexual intimacy. His wife, in turn, interprets this as a sign of rejection and as a confirmation of her own fears that she is no longer sexually attractive. It is important that the husband and wife communicate with each other about all their emotions, including their feelings about sex. In general, resuming a satisfactory sexual relationship will help a woman to recover psychologically and also may be a sign that she is doing well emotionally. If a woman does not feel ready to resume her previous level of sexuality, it is frequently helpful for her at least to have a warm and tender relationship with her partner, one of caring and affection.

The situation is somewhat more difficult for the unmarried woman. If she has a partner, my advice is the same as for the married woman: to start having sex again as soon as she and her partner feel physically and emotionally ready to do so.

Some women who develop breast cancer have not had intercourse for many years and are not interested in doing so. They should obviously heed their own feelings about their physical and emotional needs. If they were not interested in sex before the mastectomy, it is unlikely that they will have any interest following surgery.

A situation that may provoke significant difficulties is one in which a single woman who has breast cancer does not have a supportive relationship with a man, but wants to have such a relationship. If a woman is eventually to become involved in a successful relationship, she must first restore her own self-image, since it is certainly difficult to develop a fulfilling relationship with others when you don't feel good about yourself. Most single women who have had breast cancer seem to feel that it is appropriate to tell their dates about their breast cancer only at the point at which they have already developed a warm and caring relationship. They feel that it is not appropriate to tell men who they hardly know. Obviously, individuals and situations vary. You must get a sense of what seems right for you.

In general, the ability to return to her former physical

and emotional relationships is a good indicator that a woman is making a healthy emotional recovery. These fulfilling relationships also help to enhance the speed and level of recovery.

CHAPTER XIV

For the Spouse
and the Family

Someone you love, one of the most important people in your life, has just learned she has breast cancer. She is in shock and needs your support to help her cope. You want to be there for her, to cushion the blow, to help her through the trauma. Yet you yourself are going through the trauma as well. You may be afraid of the future, wondering how you will respond to the serious illness and possibly even the death of someone who is so dear to you.

A woman's breast cancer may have a similar emotional impact upon each family member and loved one as it has on the woman herself. It may affect the individuals in the family, their interaction with the patient, and their interaction with one another. Each family member may be suffering emotional stress and require support, just as the patient does. Even though you want to be a source of strength and help to someone you love, you may need a shoulder on which to lean. And you may feel a bit ashamed of yourself for having any needs and fears of your own at a time when you know that your role should be one of support.

It is important that you realize it is normal for you to be having this wide range of emotions and thoughts. This is a time of trauma for your loved one, but precisely because you love her so much, it is a time of emotional upheaval for you as well, and the pressure of feeling you must be a source of strength can make that upheaval still harder to take.

The first thing you must do is to accept your own feelings without guilt. Your anxieties and the thoughts they produce are neither abnormal, atypical, nor wrong. They are the emotions that have been evoked by the trauma that is affecting your loved one, and therefore affecting you as well.

Your role now should be one of helping the person you love to cope with her illness in the most positive way. We will examine some of the elements involved in doing that, and some of the obstacles to be overcome.

One potentially major obstacle is the woman's own response to her disease. It is not uncommon for a person to respond to serious illness with hostility. She may become angry that she has been afflicted and ask, "Why me?" This hostility is frequently misdirected: though she is angry at the world in general, the patient lashes out at those closest to her. Obviously, it is important that, no matter how painful it can be, you must realize that the hostility is not truly directed toward you, but toward her victimization by the disease. Do your best to diffuse the hostility, rather than to respond with hurt anger.

Another common response of a woman who has learned that she has breast cancer is withdrawal; she may attempt to shut out the world, including her family and friends. Despite her silence, you must help her slowly to communicate. Help her express her feelings, fears, and needs. It is, of course, much easier to help her through this time of crisis if she will express to you what she is thinking, so that you can discuss her problems and assist her in working them through. Once a woman with breast cancer becomes able to articulate her concerns, and can communicate her needs to a loving, supportive person, she often begins to recover emotionally. If you can be patiently supportive even though you may feel either shut out or unfairly attacked, your loved one will probably become able to communicate with you again. It takes time and loving support, and it certainly can be frustrating.

Toward what end should the goals and efforts of family and friends be directed? Ultimately, the woman who has had breast cancer should be encouraged to resume her life, understanding that, though she has had a serious illness, she can be cured and return to her normal role. This obviously sounds simplistic, but it may be extremely difficult to achieve. Still, the reason most cancer patients are willing to undergo the discomforts of therapy is that they want to live and they believe they have many things to live for. They have been willing to suffer the traumas of therapy in exchange for a chance to claim the pleasures of life. It makes sense, therefore, that they truly wish to believe they can be returned to the state of good physical and emotional health that they enjoyed before they developed breast cancer.

So, as soon as they are physically able, women who have been treated for breast cancer should be encouraged to resume their normal activities. (Of course, the doctor must be a guide as to when a woman is ready for each particular step.)

In general, particularly for women who enjoy their jobs, I think that the cancer patient should be encouraged to return to work as soon as she is able to do so. Work is an integral part of life for many people and adds an important element to their well-being. Returning to work may also be a symbol, a sign, to the woman that she can continue to be the same person as before the surgery. Family members should be encouraging and supportive of her decision to return to work.

One way people try to show their devotion and concern for the former patient is by paying special attention to her and performing many of the chores for which she was previously responsible. To some extent, this exhibits to the woman that her family and friends want to be supportive, and can be quite helpful. However, I have seen it carried to extremes, to the point where the woman felt she was being treated as an invalid. Uncommonly solicitous behavior may cause a woman to worry inappropriately that she must be extremely ill if her husband, who previously wouldn't empty the garbage, is now cooking six-course meals, and her daughter, who wouldn't throw her socks in the hamper, now does the laundry twice a day. It is important that you express your love, attentiveness, and willingness to give of yourself, but you must make certain that your expressions are perceived as love and support rather than as a sign that your loved one has become a hopeless invalid.

Besides encouraging her to resume her career and her daily routines, you should also encourage the woman who has been treated for breast cancer to resume her social life as soon as she is able. Take her to the movies, out to dinner, or even to a small party, when she and her doctor feel she is well enough to go. Once she realizes that her family has not abandoned her in her time of crisis, the next hurdle is for her to be reassured that her friends still have the same feelings toward her. Visiting in the hospital and sending gifts and flowers are important, but they are activities directed by a healthy person toward a sick one; however, socializing as equals carries a different connotation. If you always played bridge together, do so again; if you always went to dinner together, go out together again. The woman will feel no longer that healthy people are visiting her as an obligation but, rather, that she has resumed social relationships with friends. When this occurs, it is important that you treat her as you always did. Don't tiptoe around her.

The resumption of sexual relations is another step that reassures many women who have had breast cancer that they are once again well. Yet this is an event that the woman frequently approaches with some trepidation.

It is common for a woman who has been treated for breast cancer, particularly if she has had a mastectomy, to worry that she is no longer sexually desirable. She wants reassurance from her lover in both subtle and overt ways. But she herself is frequently quite hesitant to discuss resuming sex or to initiate sexual intimacy.

Her partner, on the other hand, may also be unsure about what to do. He is afraid that he may harm his wife physically if he initiates intercourse too soon after the surgery. He knows that he must be careful of her chest wall and of her arm on the affected side. He also knows that she has been through a great trauma and that she has been under stress and that she may not yet be emotionally ready for sexual relations.

Unfortunately, frequently because each partner is so cautious of the other's feelings at this time, trying to second-guess what is going on in the other's psyche, weeks may turn into months as the partners remain fearful of approaching each other. In the meantime, the wife has become increasingly convinced that her husband no longer finds her desirable and the husband has become convinced that the trauma of the surgery has caused his wife to lose interest in sex. Obviously, this sexual miscommunication or lack of communication may further stress a relationship that has already been seriously stressed by the trauma of the illness.

There are ways to avoid this sexual miscommunication. To start with, sexual intimacy does not necessarily require coitus. Kissing, cuddling, hugging, and fondling are romantic and intimate gestures. You can show that you still find your wife desirable very shortly after surgery by sharing these intimate gestures with her, even though you may both realize that you will not be truly sexually active for many weeks. By sharing this sense of intimacy, you will make it more likely that, when your wife *is* physically ready to have sex again, it will seem natural for you both and the transition will be easier.

You have encouraged your wife to believe that she should consider herself a woman who has had breast cancer but who is now well in all ways and should resume all the aspects of her life that she took pleasure in before her illness. You have helped her to feel healthy and whole once again. However, it is also essential that you encourage her to keep exactly to her appointment schedule and postoperative-care plan. If she requires chemotherapy, make sure she adheres to her treatment schedule. Don't let her miss her follow-up appointments or her scheduled X-ray studies. It is imperative that she do all that can be done to stay healthy, and you may well have to encourage her to make certain she does follow the plan her doctor has worked out. If she is reluctant to keep her appointments, go with her. This will serve both to make sure that she is receiving her required care and to reassure her of your support and concern.

It is obvious that breast cancer affects a woman's interactions with each of her family members as well as with her personal friends and her colleagues at work. What is frequently overlooked is that breast cancer has a far-reaching impact and may set off a cascade of changes in a series of relationships, frequently affecting the entire dynamics of a family. For instance, if a woman with breast cancer reacts by withdrawing from her husband and children, this will obviously result in tension in those particular relationships. In addition, this may subsequently stress the relationship of the husband with the children. The stress at home may in turn affect each family member's performance at work or school and relationships with peers. Family members must be aware of this possibility and work to counteract it. Go to the source and deal with the primary problem rather than allowing it to pervade all your other relationships and aspects of life.

The impact of a malignancy on most people is such that things will never be quite the same as they were before. Often the trauma of a malignancy shocks a patient into the realization of her own mortality. In soap operas, this causes people to correct all the wrongs of their lives. They repair old misunderstandings, reunite with their previously abandoned families, make amends for the social ills of their lives, and emerge victorious. But in real life, malignancy does not have such a cathartic effect on most people. It would be unrealistic to think that all people derive wisdom and happiness from surviving the trauma.

However, your goal, as the family of a woman who has been treated for a malignancy, should be to help her to emerge feeling as emotionally whole as she was prior to her illness. She has been ill, but that was in the past. She must now resume all the joys of her life that she experienced before—her family, career, friends, and special interests. Your challenge is to help her understand that she is the same human being, equally beautiful, equally productive and useful, and equally loved.

CHAPTER XV

After Treatment— the Future

You have undergone the trauma of hearing the diagnosis and of having therapy. You have withstood these pains for a purpose. Your goal now is to return to your life— not only the daily business of living, but also the especially pleasurable aspects of life. The statistics are encouraging; they show that chances are good that you will now lead a long and healthy life. Make that life enjoyable. Work through the crisis of your illness, resolve the problems that it has caused as best you can, and pick up where you left off.

Millions of women who have had breast cancer have returned to pleasurable, exciting, fruitful lives. Others have let the thought of their disease overwhelm them so that, though they were physically cured of their malignancy, they remained psychologically haunted by the disease and never resumed the life that was awaiting them.

Obviously, the stress of developing breast cancer is enormous, and it is not easy to put that behind you and go on. You must make major psychological adjustments. You must resolve the impact that the disease has upon your family. Physical adjustment may require considerable effort as well. But it would be a tragedy to let the specter of malignancy destroy your life or become your main focus. Instead, realize that there are many traumas in life, that you are fortunate enough to be in remission, and that you have a great deal to look forward to.

An excellent program that helps women adjust to their new circumstances following breast cancer is the Reach to Recovery program. Reach to Recovery was founded in 1952 by Terese Lasser, a mastectomy patient who felt that there was much that could be done to help a woman to adjust to her breast surgery, and that there was a gap between the needs of these women and what was actually being provided. Reach to Recovery merged with the American Cancer Society in 1969. The program has more than ten thousand trained volunteers who have had breast cancer, and who are now helping other women to approach their lives with a positive attitude. Once the attending surgeon has given written permission, sometimes only a few days following surgery, the Reach to Recovery volunteer visits the patient to offer help. These volunteers have all had breast cancer themselves. They are carefully screened and well trained so that they can provide appropriate help and support. The program tries to match the patient with a volunteer of approximately the same age and background. Besides providing a great deal of practical assistance, the volunteer is an excellent role model. The patient can look at and speak with her and realize that here is a woman who has been through the same trauma and who was able to put her life back together successfully. The Reach to Recovery program is also excellent for the volunteers, since they realize how much they have to give and what a great contribution they can make to the lives of others.

The diagnosis and treatment of a malignancy always has a profound effect upon a person's life, and if a woman has breast cancer, particularly if she is treated by mastectomy, the psychological impact may be devastating. Soon after a mastectomy, patients may have a sense of loss and of disbelief. It is shocking to look at the scar and to touch it, yet the woman must. Before going on with her life, she must accept what has happened, including the loss of the breast, if that was part of her treatment.

Shortly after a mastectomy, a patient can use a temporary prosthesis, a lightweight bra filled with gauze and worn over the surgical dressing. Later on, she can obtain a permanent prosthesis sized and weighted to match her other breast. Artificial nipples are also made and can be worn with the breast prosthesis. For women who want to wear something to bed, a lighter, more comfortable prosthesis is available. Breast prostheses are expensive. Some people have insurance that will pay for them. Have your doctor write a prescription.

Another thing to expect after having a mastectomy is that you will be advised to perform special exercises in the early postoperative period. These should be done only as advised by your doctor and will require medical supervision. Supervised postmastectomy exercise is important to help you retain strength in the muscles of the arm and hand and a normal amount of shoulder movement.

A woman must be very careful to protect her arm on the side of the mastectomy. One problem that may occur is lymphedema, a swelling and collection of fluid in that arm. This can be treated with arm elevation, a low-salt diet, an elastic sleeve to reduce the accumulation of fluid, and antibiotics if infection is present. However, you may be able to prevent lymphedema by following your physician's instructions properly and exercising great care.

A woman who has had a mastectomy must avoid using the arm on the affected side for heavy work. She must never constrict the arm with clothing, a shoulder bag, or a tight watch. She must never have blood drawn or her blood pressure taken on the affected side, and must avoid injury to and infection of the arm and hand. She should not hold a cigarette in that hand and must be very careful not to get burned when cooking. She must not get a sunburn, but should tan gradually. If the arm becomes swollen, tender, hot, or red, or if she has any other difficulty, she should consult her doctor immediately.

After mastectomy, because of the transient depression which some women experience, they may start to gain weight or disregard their grooming. It is important to go on taking care of your personal appearance. Knowing that you can still look and feel attractive is important.

Women may need to alter their wardrobes to some extent following a mastectomy. They may need to buy clothing with a different cut, although with some imagination, women often find that with minor modification they can continue to use most of their existing wardrobe. Women often need to buy special bathing suits. There are stores that cater to women who have had a mastectomy, selling special bathing suits, underwear, and other needed items. It is important not to skimp on such things: the money you spend on them is money you're investing in helping yourself to look and feel attractive.

Following therapy, women should try to return to their usual activities as soon as the doctor says it is reasonable to do so. Family and social activities should be resumed. Unless the patient has special reasons for not wishing or being able to do so, I think it is a good idea for previously working women to return to work. One concern that a cancer patient may have regards job discrimination. Fortunately, some states now have laws prohibiting discrimination against employees because they have or previously had a malignancy. In states without such employment protection laws, lawyers have fought against job discrimination for cancer patients by referring to the laws that prevent job discrimination against the disabled. It is important for both the woman affected and her employer to realize that, although she has had cancer, her chances of being cured of the disease are quite good, particularly if the tumor was diagnosed early. In most instances, women who have been treated for breast cancer should ultimately be able to return to work with little or no difficulty. There may be some exceptions, depending on the nature of the job and the type of treatment required.

Careful follow-up by your doctor is important. The physician will be evaluating you regularly, both for the possibility of recurrent cancer and also for the possibility of a new cancer in the other breast. Although careful, regular physical examination cannot prevent either of these problems, they do make it considerably more likely that, should a woman develop a new or recurrent tumor, there will be the greatest opportunity to find it as early as possible, enhancing her chances of being completely cured.

The recommended frequency and intervals for follow-up visits will vary somewhat from doctor to doctor and will also be somewhat dependent upon the individual needs of each patient. Follow-up visits may be about every three months for the first two years and every four to six months thereafter. Since breast cancer can recur well over ten years following the primary tumor, and the other breast always remains at increased risk, women must continue to be evaluated throughout their lives.

At each visit the doctor will take a thorough history of any problems the woman has encountered since she was last in the office. Then she will have a careful physical examination. She will also need to have periodic blood studies, chest X-rays, mammography, and possibly bone scans.

In some circumstances, a physician might feel that scans of the liver or brain would be helpful, to make sure the cancer has not recurred. None of these studies are painful, and in certain instances they may be quite useful.

Besides keeping her regular appointments, the woman who has been treated for breast cancer must be alert to certain problems and let her doctor know immediately if they occur. She should be doing monthly breast self-examination and report any abnormal findings to her physician. She should consult her physician if she develops hoarseness, a persistent cough, new digestive difficulties, or bone pain. She should also consult the doctor if she finds any new swellings or lumps or anything potentially suggestive of tumor.

It is unreasonable and unproductive for the woman who has been treated for breast cancer to go through life with a cloud over her head, constantly fearful of the potential for recurrent disease. On the other hand, if she has abnormal findings, she must pay attention to them. Recurrent breast cancer may be curable, but it must be treated immediately to ensure the best chances for success.

In summary, developing breast cancer and being treated for it are clearly major traumas for a woman to sustain. Reaching full emotional and psychological recovery may require great effort. Women must try as much as possible not to let the disease remain the major focus of their lives. It is encouraging to realize that hundreds of thousands of women have been able to return to happy, satisfying, productive lives after being treated for the disease.

CHAPTER XVI

Living
with Breast Cancer

Throughout this book, I have stressed that breast cancer is a curable disease, and that most women who have breast cancer can be restored to good health, particularly if they seek therapy early in the course of the illness. I have encouraged women to attempt to resume their lives with positive energy once the disease has been diagnosed and they have undergone therapy. I urge the woman who has been treated for breast cancer to enjoy her life, living fully, assuming she will be among the large number whose primary therapy results in cure.

Yet, unfortunately, for some women, their breast cancer will recur, and, of course, almost all women to whom this happens feel devastated and frightened. If a breast cancer recurs, the woman will experience many of the same emotions she had when she learned of her original tumor, but they may be even harder to take.

As I have said throughout, it is essential that a woman who has had breast cancer receive follow-up screening according to the exact guidelines outlined by her doctor, undergoing the designated tests and reporting any abnormal symptoms. Avoiding follow-up testing and failing to report abnormal symptoms will not prevent the recurrence of breast cancer. Denying that breast cancer can recur can delay diagnosis and required therapy and impair the ultimate outcome for the woman.

I encourage women who have had cancer to regard themselves, once therapy has been completed, as treated, to put the disease in the past, and to resume their lives as positively and pleasurably as possible. But they must also realize that follow-up is necessary, a means of staying healthy rather than a harbinger of illness.

Depending on the extent of the primary disease, the initial therapy, and subsequent findings, prescribed follow-up may include chest X-rays, blood studies, bone scans, bone X-rays, mammography, and less commonly liver scans and CT scans. In the future, as the technology and expertise are further refined, NMR (nuclear magnetic resonance imaging) may be used more frequently. Physical examination by the physician is, of course, an important part of the follow-up plan.

The woman who has had breast cancer will also be examining herself, continuing to perform breast self-examination on the remaining breast if she has had a mastectomy, or on both breasts if she has had a tylectomy and radiation therapy. If she has had a mastectomy, she should be alert for any nodules in the area of the scar, or on the chest wall in the area of the mastectomy. She should also look for any enlargement of lymph nodes, particularly in the underarm or above the clavicle (collar bone). If a woman who has been treated for breast cancer notes any of these possibly abnormal findings, she should immediately tell her doctor.

Some findings that may indicate a recurrence of the disease are difficult to distinguish from other, minor problems, totally unrelated to the breast cancer. They should, in general, be reported to the doctor, so that he or she can determine whether they do represent a significant problem.

Caution is one thing—and, as I have said repeatedly, a vital one for the woman who has had breast cancer—but it is unfortunate and counterproductive when a person is so overly fearful of developing a recurrent malignancy that each ache or pain becomes a major psychological trauma. It is, of course, difficult for people to change their behavior patterns. Many people will be overly fearful of developing a recurrence and will become alarmed each time they develop any minor problem. This is more common immediately after a breast cancer has been treated. Over time, fear and anxiety lessen, and this behavior usually diminishes. On the other hand, some people will deny that they might develop a recurrence and will ignore what are clearly serious problems. The obvious answer lies in striking a balance between these harmful extremes.

It is difficult to change a person's nature. By the time a woman reaches the age when she might develop a breast malignancy, she is quite set in her habits and has a relatively personal and fixed way of responding to crises. For some people, this may be almost as individual and unalterable as their fingerprints. There is, fortunately, one way to change a patient's response to possible symptoms that occur following therapy for breast cancer: detailed conversation with a physician or a counselor regarding exactly what symptoms the woman should be alert to. In my years of caring for women who have had malignancies, I have found that many women are simply not aware of exactly what they should be concerned about.

After a woman has been treated for breast cancer, her doctor will probably describe to her in detail the symptoms that might be suggestive of recurrence and should be reported immediately. For most women, this conversation may take place prematurely. A woman who has just been through her initial therapy for breast cancer has so many more immediate concerns, both medical and social, not to mention her psychological needs. She is digesting so much information pertaining to her present condition that it is unlikely that she can also fully incorporate information on what's important in the distant future.

I feel, therefore, that several months after the initial therapy for breast cancer, the patient should review, either with her physician or with a counselor, exactly which problems should cause her concern and be reported. If the doctor feels that the patient is continuing either to overreact or to deny, or if the patient continues to feel uncertain about what may represent true and significant symptoms, this conversation can be repeated at appropriate intervals, as the woman has her regular follow-up appointments.

Although I believe that this is really the province of the medical team that is providing care for the woman, and that any conversations between a woman and her doctor are specific to her needs and therefore take precedence over anything that applies to a general group of women, the following is a list of some of the symptoms that should cause a woman who has had breast cancer to contact her physician:

1. A persistent cough. A woman who has had breast cancer can get a cold just like any other person, and each sneeze should not be the cause of a major psychological trauma. However, a persistent cough, particularly in the absence of a cold, may be indicative of a recurrence of disease in the lungs.

2. A significant weight loss. Although the loss of a few pounds is usually not cause for concern, the

loss of a considerable amount of weight may be a manifestation of a real problem.

3. Gastrointestinal symptoms, such as loss of appetite, abdominal bloating, cramping, persistent nausea and vomiting, or a persistent change in bowel habits. Most people periodically have some kind of gastrointestinal distress. They may eat or drink too much at a party and experience the consequences for the next day or two. A common minor medical problem that some people refer to as the twenty-four-hour flu or intestinal virus may result in a short interval of nausea and vomiting and an inability to eat or drink. These common medical problems affect most people from time to time, including those who have had breast cancer. In general, they represent no cause for alarm.

In contrast to these relatively harmless disturbances, other types of bowel symptoms may indeed indicate a recurrence of cancer in the abdomen. These gastrointestinal problems are usually of a more indolent nature: their onset is usually gradual and the difficulties persist. People who develop a recurrent malignancy in the abdomen may note that over a period of time their appetite lessens and they develop a sensation of abdominal bloating. They may also have a sensation of abdominal cramping, which may increase in severity after meals. Chronic nausea may occur, ultimately with vomiting. A persistent change in bowel habits may be noted.

Though the symptoms just described may be of significance and should be evaluated by the doctor, isolated episodes of abdominal problems following overeating or short-term viral infection must be kept in perspective.

4. Bone pain. The bones are a common location for recurrent or metastatic breast cancer. Therefore, persistent bone pain must be reported to the doctor and will almost always require evaluation. Alternatively, most people do bump and bruise themselves periodically, causing some short-term discomfort. Mild pain that occurs as a result of a minor accident should not immediately be taken to mean that metastatic breast cancer is present. If you relax and wait a few days, the discomfort may disappear. If it doesn't, call your doctor.

5. Other pain. Pain in general may be an indication of significant disease; if it is persistent, it should be evaluated by the physician.

6. Nodules, lumps, and masses. These usually require a medical examination and may need to be biopsied. Lesions of particular concern include those on or under the skin, those near the site of the previous surgical scar, those in the other breast, or those in the affected breast if a lumpectomy and radiation therapy were performed. The enlargement of lymph nodes, particularly under the arm, in the neck, or above the clavicle, may be an indication of recurrent disease. It is important that these lumps not be ignored. They should be evaluated immediately by the doctor, for they may quite possibly be signs of recurrent disease. If either a local recurrence or a new cancer in the other breast is evaluated and diagnosed early, and treated promptly, the outcome is likely to be good.

7. Inappropriate bleeding. Hemoptysis (coughing up blood), hematemesis (vomiting blood), hematuria (blood in the urine), and blood in the stool may each be an indication of a serious problem—whether related to the previous breast cancer or not. Any one of these problems should be reported to the physician. Further evaluation will probably be warranted.

8. Neurological problems. Double vision, blurred vision, chronic headaches, and other neurological symptoms must be evaluated.

9. General malaise. This is hard to evaluate adequately. Some people who have undergone therapy for a malignancy have a sense of fatigue or chronic illness that is based in depression brought on by the illness, or in other psychological problems. Yet general malaise and fatigue may also be indicators of recurrent tumor. Both should be reported to the doctor: whatever the cause, they can and should be evaluated and treated.

The aforementioned discussion has reviewed many of the types of findings that may be significant for the individual who has previously been treated for breast cancer. It is important to strike a balance between undue alarm, which may be psychologically counterproductive, and flippant denial, which may be medically dangerous. I have cared for women who have been treated for malignancy who almost daily find a new frightening symptom, living in constant fear that they will develop a recurrent malignancy. Although I can fully understand and sympathize with their fears, it saddens me to have them suffer such unnecessary pain. They have already suffered with the illness and with its therapy. The excessive fear of recurrence usually causes a serious erosion in the quality of life for these women. I am frequently able to allay their anxieties to some degree, and I believe that a serious conversation with a supportive physician can put the reality of physical symptoms and anxiety-generated symptoms into perspective.

Again it is important that the woman who has had breast cancer carefully review with her physician which symptoms the doctor considers of potential concern and which he or she feels require especially prompt attention, given the individual woman's specific problems. I cannot underscore sufficiently the fact that all breast cancers and all individuals are not uniform, and that communication between the woman and her doctor regarding potential sources of concern is essential.

What happens when the symptoms a woman finds do in fact signify the presence of a recurrent malignancy? First, a very thorough evaluation will be done to determine whether this represents an isolated focus of recurrent disease or whether the tumor is present in several sites. The doctor will perform a complete physical examination and obtain several blood studies, and may order some of the following radiologic studies: a chest X-ray, bone X-rays, a mammography of the other breast (and the originally affected breast, if it was not removed as part of the primary therapy), a bone scan, a liver scan, a brain scan, a CT scan (computerized tomography, a very sensitive method of evaluating individual organs and cross-sections of the body for relatively small foci of disease), and possibly NMR (nuclear magnetic resonance imaging, a technique in which the body is exposed to a magnetic field to evaluate the presence of tumor masses). In many instances, a biopsy will be necessary to make absolutely sure that the findings do actually represent recurrent tumor.

What to expect once a recurrence has been diagnosed will depend upon the site of the cancer. It is very important to realize that recurrent disease can be treated and that many thousands of women who have had recurrent breast cancer are living their lives quite comfortably, normally, and actively.

One of the locations in which breast cancer may commonly recur is on the site of the scar or the chest wall itself. This may be treated locally first, with surgery or radiation therapy. Subsequently, a systemic therapy—chemotherapy or hormonal treatment—may be advised. Women who develop a local recurrence at the site of their previous surgery have a better prognosis than patients who develop metastatic disease in other areas of the body. Many women who develop recurrent disease at the scar or on the chest wall will be alive five years later.

As is discussed extensively in chapter VI, many women are now electing to have as their primary therapy for breast cancer a lumpectomy and lymph node removal followed by radiation, without removal of the breast. We are finding that some of these women are developing recurrent cancer within the breast tissue that has been preserved. In almost all instances when this happens, the women do require mastectomy. Since there is not a large body of data available on long-term survival for women who have been treated with lumpectomy and radiation therapy, it is not absolutely clear what cure rate can be expected for the woman whose breast cancer has been treated with primary radiation therapy and who develops a recurrence in the breast and is subsequently treated with mastectomy. There are some data that suggest that the chances of cure for such women will be good, but there is not yet sufficient proof for us to be completely certain.

The bones are another site at which breast cancer commonly recurs, as stated earlier. The return of breast cancer in the bones may show up either with bone pain or as a fracture. If a recurrence in the bone is found, it is, again, important to determine whether it represents an isolated focus of disease, or whether the bone disease was just the first manifestation of widespread recurrent tumor. Radiation may be used to treat one or more isolated areas of bone metastases, particularly if the areas are painful. Patients who have bone metastases will probably require systemic therapy. Although the prognosis is not as good for the patient with bone metastases as it is for the woman who has an isolated recurrence in the breast or at the site of the previous surgery, several women who have developed bone recurrences have been alive and living well five years later.

Other possible sites of recurrent tumor include the lung, abdominal cavity, liver, and brain. In general, recurrent disease in these sites does not have as favorable an outcome as recurrence in the chest wall, breast, skin, scar, or bone. Patients who have recurrent disease in these areas of poorer prognosis may initially be treated with surgery and/or radiation therapy, particularly if the tumor is found only in a single area. However, systemic therapy is essential for the woman with such serious recurrent disease.

As I discussed previously, thousands of women who have been treated for recurrent breast cancer live comfortably and normally. Clearly, developing recurrent breast cancer is a frightening event, perhaps even more traumatic than the original cancer. However, a woman who has had the courage to cope with the primary tumor, and to realize that she can return to a happy and productive life, will usually be able to call forth her inner strength once again if a recurrence does develop.

If breast cancer recurs, there should be an emphasis on

maximizing the quality of life. Whereas cure following the recurrence of breast cancer is less likely, comfortable long-term remissions lasting many years frequently occur. This makes it essential that if there is a recurrence and if conventional medical therapies that are known to be able to provide control are available, these therapies be evaluated for the individual and used appropriately.

It is vital for the woman who develops recurrent breast cancer to realize that she has a treatable problem that can usually be controlled. Otherwise, even if the woman is free of disease for many years, she will not enjoy the psychological comfort that would help to make her life more satisfying.

CHAPTER XVII

Breast Cancer and Pregnancy

In past generations, breast cancer occurring simultaneously with pregnancy was a relatively uncommon event. I expect that, given current alterations in life styles in our society, it may happen more commonly in the future. Why is this? We know that a woman's likelihood of developing breast cancer increases if she does not have a baby during her early to middle years of fertility. We also know that the risk of developing breast cancer increases as women age. It is becoming increasingly common to see women in their later thirties or even their early forties who are having a first child. These women are obviously at greater risk of developing breast cancer during pregnancy than a twenty-five-year-old pregnant woman, by virtue of their age and their postponement of childbearing.

Because breast cancer occurring during pregnancy was a relatively uncommon event in past generations, there is a lot that we do not yet know about the best approach to the problem.

Two distinct considerations must be addressed when a pregnant woman develops breast cancer: what are the effects of the pregnancy on the breast cancer, and what are the effects of the breast cancer on the pregnancy and the baby? Breast cancer is always a devastating illness, but it is even more so when the physical and emotional stresses of being diagnosed and treated are complicated by pregnancy.

Most studies indicate that, at any given stage of the disease, the prognosis for the breast cancer patient will be the same whether or not she is pregnant. However, most reports in which large numbers of pregnant women are evaluated do show that the likelihood of a woman's being cured if she develops breast cancer during pregnancy is quite poor. The explanation for this apparent paradox is that, when a woman is diagnosed as having breast cancer during pregnancy, she is likely to have more extensive disease.

When a woman is pregnant, her breasts usually become larger and engorged, and there may be more flow of blood and lymph. This increased flow may cause a more rapid dissemination of tumor to the lymphatics (channels that carry fluid and cells to lymph nodes). In addition, since the breasts do change so much during pregnancy, it may be more difficult for a woman or her doctor to diagnose a malignancy until the tumor is larger. And screening mammography (which is often used to evaluate seemingly normal breasts, in order to detect tumors too small to be felt by the woman or her doctor) is not performed during pregnancy unless a mass is felt.

In general, women perceive pregnancy to be a time of good health, a positive and happy experience. They may find it difficult to believe that a lump they feel in their breast could be anything but another change brought on by their normal pregnancy. A woman may thus note a suspicious mass but be reluctant to mention it to her doctor, delaying the discovery of a possible malignancy.

What are the problems encountered in treating breast cancer during pregnancy? Technically, the various types of surgery that might be performed for a woman with breast cancer are probably not much more difficult whether or not she is pregnant. There might be a bit more bleeding because of the increased blood flow to the breast. Although the chances that the anesthetic or the surgery will have a negative effect on the pregnancy are not extremely high, there is some risk that the procedure could result in a miscarriage or in premature labor.

Most radiation therapists seem to feel that radiation therapy to the breast should not be given during pregnancy because of the risks to the fetus. Even if an attempt is made to use a lead shield for protection, safety to the offspring cannot be assured.

Women with breast cancer are frequently advised to have chemotherapy. There is a growing body of information available on the use of chemotherapy during pregnancy. In general, chemotherapy affects tissues that are most rapidly growing, and the pre-natal development of a fetus is clearly a time of very rapid growth. Chemotherapy is extremely toxic to a fetus during the early stages of pregnancy, at which time its use is more likely to result in malformation or miscarriage. During the latter stages of pregnancy, some drugs are considered more dangerous to the fetus than others. For instance, Methotrexate, a chemotherapeutic agent used in many breast-cancer regimens, should not be given to a pregnant woman unless her circumstances are dire. Although a variety of factors must be considered, unless the situation is quite urgent, chemotherapists prefer to wait until a woman has her baby before using chemotherapy.

One enormous decision facing a woman who is diagnosed as having breast cancer while she is pregnant is whether or not to terminate the pregnancy.

Some doctors feel that the pregnancy does not in itself hasten the growth of the malignancy, and that having an abortion does not necessarily improve the prognosis under typical conditions. However, if keeping the pregnancy makes a woman unable or unwilling to receive a certain beneficial therapy, abortion might improve her chances of cure. Another consideration is that breast cancer in general appears to be a hormonally dependent tumor, and hormone levels are extremely high during pregnancy. Therefore, the high levels of circulating hormones present during pregnancy could theoretically cause breast cancer to grow rapidly if the pregnancy is not terminated.

Furthermore, as discussed earlier, the cure rates for breast cancer diagnosed during pregnancy are considerably poorer than those for breast cancer diagnosed in a nonpregnant woman. Although it is frightening to face this issue, a woman in such a situation must realize that her baby might have a very sick mother or no mother at all to help in its upbringing.

If breast cancer is diagnosed early in a pregnancy, at a stage when abortion is legal and safe, many factors must be considered in deciding whether to terminate the pregnancy. The woman must make sure that she has discussed fully with her doctor all the potential risks, to herself and to the baby.

A woman whose breast cancer is diagnosed when she is carrying a pregnancy that has progressed beyond the twenty-fourth week, making abortion out of the question, is usually treated for her breast cancer in a manner that is as safe as possible for the baby. If chemotherapy or radiation is thought to be potentially beneficial for the patient, and if it is thought that the baby is probably mature enough to be delivered, the physician may advise a premature delivery. This will enable the chemotherapy or radiation to be given without having any potential effects on the baby. If breast cancer is diagnosed in the latter part of pregnancy and the woman requires surgery alone as therapy, many doctors consider it acceptable to perform the surgery and then just permit the patient to go into a normal labor and have a normal delivery when the time comes.

If a woman who has breast cancer does continue with her pregnancy, the possibility of transmitting the cancer to the offspring is minuscule. (Of course, if the baby is a girl, she is statistically at high risk of developing breast cancer when she becomes an adult, since her mother had breast cancer at an early age.)

If a woman who has been treated for breast cancer during pregnancy does continue the pregnancy, I think that it is preferable that she bottle-feed the newborn rather than breast-feed. When a woman breast-feeds, there are theoretical possibilities both of transmitting a carcinogen to the baby via the milk, or worsening the course of her own disease due to the high hormone levels present during lactation.

Since many women are now choosing to delay having their families until they are older, the question of whether and when it is reasonable for a woman previously treated for breast cancer to consider becoming pregnant will arise more and more frequently. The answer to this varies considerably, depending on the woman's individual circumstances. The physical aspects of the tumor are important— its size, the involvement of lymph nodes or other locations of metastases, the presence of estrogen and progesterone receptors, etc. In addition, how old a woman is and whether she has any other children are factors that should be taken into consideration. The standard answer may be that a woman should wait a few years following breast cancer therapy before she considers becoming pregnant, but women who are at very high risk of developing recurrent breast cancer may be advised by their doctors never to become pregnant.

There are several reasons for the recommendation that women put off becoming pregnant for a few years, if they are interested in having another child and if they decide that the risks in their particular circumstance are reasonable. One is that breast cancers are often stimulated to grow by certain hormones that are present in substantial amounts during pregnancy. If a woman still has a few malignant cells in her body following her therapy for breast cancer, there could, theoretically, be a rapid increase in the activity of these cells if she becomes pregnant. Since many of the breast cancers that recur do so early on, waiting a few years to become pregnant might reduce the risk somewhat.

And, of course, a woman who is contemplating having a baby wants to have as much reassurance as possible that she will be able to care for and raise the child. By waiting a few years, she can at least put behind her the time when she was at greatest risk of developing an early recurrence of disease. Women who are at extremely high risk should probably not get pregnant.

The treatment of recurrent or advanced breast cancer in a young woman may involve ablation (destruction) of her ovarian function, by radiation to or removal of the ovaries. Under such circumstances, a woman would be unable to become pregnant.

Pregnancy is usually a beautiful experience, but breast cancer can turn it into a tragic one. As at all other times, women should be alert to the changes in their bodies and in their breasts. Women should continue to do monthly breast self-examination during pregnancy. A lump identified during pregnancy deserves attention as immediately as a mass found at any other time. Perhaps if breast cancer during pregnancy can be identified earlier in the course of the disease, just as we are striving to do for the nonpregnant woman with breast cancer, we can ultimately achieve a better outcome for both the woman and her family.

CHAPTER XVIII

Breast Cancer in Men

Breast cancer is considered a woman's illness, and for the most part this it true, but men do develop the disease. Approximately one percent of all breast cancers diagnosed occur in men. Although the cause of breast cancer, whether in women or men, is not yet fully understood, there is no scientific information to indicate that a man is at increased risk of developing breast cancer if he is in close contact with a woman who has the disease. In fact, it is believed that breast cancer is not transmittable from one adult to another, whether male or female.

Since women are at such high risk of developing breast cancer, they are repeatedly being advised to examine their breasts each month. In general, men have not been given such an admonition. The risk to any individual man of developing breast cancer is quite small, but it has been estimated that between .1 percent and 1.5 percent of all cancers in men originate in the breast. Therefore, periodic examination both by the man himself and by his doctor seems warranted.

Statistically, men who have breast cancer usually have a poor outcome—because breast cancer is usually not diagnosed in men until the lesion is quite advanced. Approximately one-third of the breast cancers seen in men are considered to be inoperable by the time the man first seeks help from his doctor.

The prognosis for men who have breast cancer should be improved somewhat just by informing men that they, too, can develop breast cancer and should therefore, examine themselves and be alert to any abnormal symptoms. The most common symptoms for a man who harbors a breast cancer include a palpable breast mass, a bloody discharge from the nipple, a pulling or inversion of the nipple, pain in the breast or underarm, or a mass in the underarm. If a man notices any of these signs, he should see a doctor immediately to check for breast cancer. Men who have received radiation to the breast are thereafter at greatly increased risk of developing a breast malignancy.

Breast cancer in men occurs mostly in the older age group. The average age at diagnosis is sixty. Only six percent of men's breast cancers occur in men who are under the age of forty, but cases of breast cancer have been diagnosed in boys as young as five and six.

The primary therapy for breast cancer in the male is similar to that in the female. If the lesion has not become too extensive, the initial treatment is surgery. The surgery itself seems to provoke much less psychological trauma in men than it does in women. Unfortunately, however, as I mentioned, so many of the breast cancers diagnosed in men are inoperable, because the men have ignored their symptoms for too long and allowed the cancer to become quite extensive. For advanced tumors, radiation therapy may be used. Men who have disseminated breast cancer may require orchiectomy (castration) to help control the tumor.

Although breast cancer does not occur as commonly in men as it does in women, it is clearly a problem of equally great magnitude when it does occur. If a man has an operable breast cancer, the prognosis will be the same for him as it would be for a woman who had a similar tumor. My hope is that more and more men will become alert to the fact that they too may develop breast cancer and will stop ignoring the symptoms and waiting too long to consult a doctor. It is so unfortunate when a life that could easily have been saved is lost due to a delay in diagnosis.

CHAPTER XIX

Cystic Disease

Millions of women have been told that they have cystic breasts. They worry, naturally, and repeatedly ask, "Does this mean I am at increased risk of developing breast cancer?"

There are some data indicating that the woman who truly has gross cystic disease of the breasts (classified by Dr. Cushman Haagensen, a professor of surgery at Columbia College of Physicians and Surgeons who has contributed greatly to our understanding of breast cancer, as cysts that are larger than three millimeters in diameter) is more likely to develop breast cancer later. However, the term "cystic disease" is much overused, and a significant percentage of the women who fear they suffer from this problem are mistaken. Many of them are actually just experiencing the normal changes that occur in the breasts each month, as a result of the cyclic variation in the level of hormones related to their menstrual periods.

If you examine your breasts within several days before the onset of your period, they may feel somewhat different, because of changes in hormone levels. If you repeat the examination a few days after your period ends, your breasts will probably feel normal again. This happens to many women and in most cases does not represent true gross cystic disease. You should perform breast self-examination each month, approximately seven days after the onset of your menstrual period, to prevent this confusion.

This normal physiologic change related to cyclic hormonal fluctuation is just one reason cystic disease may be overdiagnosed. The important point is that even many doctors are not in complete agreement as to what represents true cystic disease of the breasts. But since many doctors think that cystic disease is a significantly overdiagnosed condition, many women who believe they have it and are therefore at increased risk of developing breast cancer are probably not at increased risk, because they don't really have true cystic disease.

On the other hand, true gross cystic disease may actually place the woman at higher risk of developing invasive breast cancer. When a woman palpates a mass in her breast, even if she believes that it is just a cyst, she should consult her doctor immediately. If a cyst is present and there is no suggestion of malignancy, the physician will usually recommend aspiration (putting a needle in the cyst and withdrawing the fluid). Whether anything further is necessary will depend upon the results of this procedure.

In some cases the doctor will determine that the woman does not have any type of cyst or mass, merely the normal physiologic changes that can occur in the premenstrual phase of the cycle. Even so, the physician will almost always want to repeat the examination later on, after the menses, to be certain that a significant mass has not been overlooked.

Some women have monthly breast symptoms shortly before the onset of their period. Once a physician has ruled out the possibility of a serious breast mass, several things can be done to alleviate this problem. One very simple step, which is frequently quite effective, is a dietary adjustment. For many women, caffeine exacerbates premenstrual breast symptoms. These women note significant, rapid relief when they eliminate caffeine from their diet. If you have monthly breast discomfort, once your doctor has ruled out the possibility of malignancy, give yourself a three-month trial of eliminating chocolate, sodas containing caffeine, coffee, tea, and any other sources of dietary caffeine. Chances are this will reduce your symptoms. As an additional benefit, eliminating these foods from your diet is likely to have several other positive health effects, including weight reduction and diminished anxiety.

Some medications may reduce the frequency and magnitude of fibrocystic disease. There is some suggestion that women who use birth-control pills may have a reduced incidence of fibrocystic disease, but these medications may have significant side effects, and most doctors are reluctant to prescribe them just to alleviate breast symptoms. On the other hand, the woman for whom the birth-control pill is an appropriate method of contraception may find the alleviation of the discomfort of cystic breasts a welcome side benefit. An androgenic hormone, Danazol, appears to offer some relief to women with fibrocystic disease. However, because it has some of the properties seen in male hormones, it may cause unwanted side effects.

So, what should the woman who believes that she has "cystic breasts" do? The first step is to try to determine what the problem actually is. As previously noted, true gross cystic disease of the breasts is a significantly overdiagnosed condition, and many women who think they suffer from it are really just experiencing monthly variations in their breasts that are totally within the normal, expected range.

At the other extreme, it is obviously important to make absolutely certain that what is being regarded as normal physiologic breast change is not actually a misdiagnosed breast cancer. One way to avoid this potentially drastic error is to remember that you should always see your doctor right away if you find a breast mass; let him or her rule out the presence of a malignancy and determine if it represents cystic disease. If a mass is present, it should be proved benign, usually by aspiration and/or biopsy, as discussed in detail in chapter V. On the other hand, cystic disease may mimic breast cancer, and a woman whose symptoms at first suggested breast cancer may be fortunate enough to be determined, after diagnostic studies, to have cystic disease only.

So, step one in the medical care of the woman who thinks she may have cystic disease is to try to confirm that diagnosis and to rule out a malignancy.

For the woman who has monthly breast changes that cause her discomfort, the next issue to address is what can be done about it. As discussed earlier, restricting caffeine intake works for many women; oral contraceptives and Danazol therapy may have their place in selected situations.

Finally, the issue that worries most women who believe they have cystic disease is whether they are at increased risk of developing breast cancer. Fortunately, many women who believe they have cystic disease actually do not, and since they have a "nondisease," they are not among the group at increased risk. On the other hand, women who have certain types of true fibrocystic disease may be at increased risk.

In any event, the approach for all these women must be the same. Those with true fibrocystic disease, overzealously diagnosed fibrocystic disease, and no fibrocystic disease essentially all require the same thing—a program of careful screening and follow-up with breast self-examination, physician examination, and mammography beginning at an appropriate age.

CHAPTER XX

Prevention

Every day, as each new patient enters my office, I discuss breast cancer screening with her. Even though I have had the same discussion thousands of times, it continues to disturb me, both as a doctor and as a woman. I hear myself saying over and over again, "As a woman in the United States, you have approximately a one-in-eleven chance of developing breast cancer. You must perform breast self-examination each month, be examined regularly by a doctor, and I advise that you participate in a program of mammography screening." The patient's risk, my risk, every woman's risk is so high. I can help a woman have her tumor diagnosed earlier. I can help save her life. But what can we as a team, the patient and I, do to prevent her from developing breast cancer?

Early detection is a laudable goal. It saves lives. It permits the option of conservative surgery, so that women can retain their breasts and still be cured of the disease. We've made great progress, but it really isn't good enough. What we truly want to be doing is preventing breast cancer. Can we do this?

Clearly, the ultimate goal of the physician in our society is to prevent disease. As a cancer surgeon, I would like nothing better than having no one who required surgery because we had become so sophisticated about preventing disease. Although this is not at present the case, we do know many things about the prevention of the disease that may be quite helpful in reducing the frequency of breast cancer.

I cannot tell you what to do in 1987 to guarantee that you will not develop breast cancer. However, thanks to the enormous increase in interest among the scientific community, the government, and the public in prevention of disease, there are many things I can tell you that are thought to be likely to decrease your risk of developing breast cancer. It is my hope that over the next several years there will be a much greater amount of definitive information on the topic. I am pleased to say that the policy of our government appears to be directed toward the expenditure of a greater percentage of medical-research funds for prevention of disease.

But what can I tell you in this book, right now, that will help you avoid ever developing a malignancy, and more specifically breast cancer? Robert McKenna, in a 1983 issue of the sophisticated and highly regarded medical journal *Cancer*, estimated that environmental factors contribute to more than eighty percent of human cancers worldwide. He estimated that in 1982 more than 125,000 malignancies in the United States alone were probably preventable had our population modified its life style.

How did he suggest that this enormous number of people could have been spared developing a malignancy? His first recommendation was the elimination of tobacco. Lung cancer appears to be surpassing breast cancer as the leading cause of cancer death among American women. It is estimated that a large proportion of such deaths could have been prevented and that these malignancies were directly related to cigarette smoking. McKenna also recommends moderation in alcohol consumption, since excessive drinking is known to contribute to cancer of the mouth, throat, and gastrointestinal tract. To editorialize, it seems so unfortunate to me that as women have continued to become more successful and have attained many of the positive professional achievements that formerly belonged within the male domain, they have adopted some destructive habits that had previously been more common among men.

McKenna also noted that the risk of malignancy can be reduced by avoiding sun exposure (which contributes to skin cancer and melanoma), avoiding carcinogenic drugs, and being cautious about X-ray exposure. He also discusses the contribution of good dietary habits and the maintenance of ideal body weight in reducing the possibility of certain types of malignancy. Because this has specific pertinence to breast cancer, I will take it up in greater detail later in this chapter.

The aforementioned are tangible ways women have immediately available to them to reduce their risk of developing a wide variety of common malignancies. Evidence has recently become apparent suggesting ways women can reduce their risk for breast cancer in particular.

To determine how we can help reduce the incidence of breast cancer and diminish any individual's risk of developing the disease, it is useful to consider the high-risk factors. By examining what features place a woman at increased risk, we can evaluate proposed scenarios to reduce this risk.

We know there is a strong hereditary component to breast cancer. A woman's risk of developing the disease increases significantly if her mother, sister, or grandmother was affected. The presence of more distant relatives who had breast cancer can also contribute to a woman's risk of developing the disease. Clearly, these hereditary factors cannot be altered.

However, there are also strong environmental and social

components to the disease, and these we can attack. We know that a Japanese woman who lives in Japan does not have a very high risk of developing breast cancer (the risk is approximately one-eighth that of a Caucasian American). However, when the Japanese family moves to the United States, succeeding generations are at greatly increased risk to develop breast cancer, so that within two generations of the move, the Japanese woman in the United States has approximately the same risk of developing breast cancer as does her Caucasian neighbor. This provides strong evidence that the environment plays a significant role in the tendency to develop breast cancer. It is postulated that the change in the diet of the Japanese family when they move to the United States contributes largely to the increased risk.

Breast cancer is, furthermore, a disease that is much more prevalent in affluent countries, and within these societies it is most likely to affect women in upper socioeconomic groups, again suggesting an environmental influence.

It is thought that one of the outstanding environmental features that increases a woman's risk of developing breast cancer is diet, a conclusion supported both by animal studies and by epidemiologic data. It has been estimated that extensive dietary modification could possibly lower the U.S. cancer death rate by as much as thirty-five percent. This is a shocking thought. All these lives lost each year, all the needless anguish, when it is likely that something as simple as modifying our diet could prevent malignancy for a large number of women.

What about the American diet is thought to increase the risk of breast cancer? The high fat content of the foods we consume appears to increase our risk greatly. How simple it would be to make this dietary modification, and, of course, to inculcate our children with better habits, too. If we feed our children healthier diets and raise them on more appropriate foods, they will come to accept these foods as their normal diet and will enjoy them as much as they now enjoy their less healthy meals and snacks.

High-fat diets seem to increase the incidence of cardiovascular disease (heart attack, stroke) and bowel malignancy as well. So this dietary modification may have many positive effects for you and your family. And a high-fat diet will contribute to obesity, which has also been linked with breast cancer, as well as with many other medical and psychological problems.

Increasing dietary fiber content by consuming more bran and fruits and vegetables is also thought to be potentially beneficial in decreasing a woman's risk of developing breast cancer. And increasing the fiber content in your diet will, like reducing your fat intake, probably decrease your susceptibility to other medical problems as well.

Having adequate vitamins in your diet is also believed to contribute to the prevention of malignancy. I am not recommending that you take megavitamins. It may be dangerous to take ultra-large doses of certain vitamins, for some cannot be excreted rapidly by the body and their buildup may produce serious side effects. What has been suggested, however, is that an appropriately balanced diet that contains essential nutrients and vitamins may help protect against malignancy.

There is evidence that vitamin A (retinoids and carotenoids) may reduce the risk of cancer and that increasing the dietary consumption of β carotene (a pigment that is converted to vitamin A in the body) may actually diminish the number of breast cancer deaths. Increased dietary consumption of vitamin C has also been postulated to offer some protection against the development of malignancy. Foods that have a high vitamin-A content include apricots, broccoli, canteloupe, carrots, spinach, peaches, pumpkin, squash, and sweet potatoes. Foods with a high vitamin-C content include broccoli, Brussels sprouts, cabbage, canteloupe, cauliflower, grapefruit, green peppers, lemons, limes, oranges, tangerines, strawberries, sweet potatoes, and tomatoes.

Knowing what I know about the possible relationship between diet and malignancy, when I dream of a luscious snack I'm much more likely to envision a bowl of fruit than I would have been five years ago, and I'm more likely to offer something appropriately healthy to my children when they're hungry. Ideas about what's delicious really are learned, and we can be teaching them to our families while we're re-educating ourselves. At present, dietary modification appears to be in the vanguard of our attempt to decrease the risk of breast cancer, as well as other malignancies and a variety of other serious illnesses.

Another issue, as I discussed earlier, revolves around the changes in recent years in our childbearing habits. A woman who is younger when she has her first child is at much less risk of developing breast cancer than one who has her first child when she is in her thirties, or who has no children at all. This fact seems unlikely to change too many decisions regarding whether and when to have children, but it is worthwhile to know.

It had been thought that women who breast-feed their children reduce their risk of developing breast cancer. Many now believe that this is probably not the case. However, there are other positive medical aspects to breast-feeding, whether or not it does decrease breast-cancer risk.

Fortunately, although some others dispute this, the Centers for Disease Control have determined that the use of the birth-control pill does not appear to increase a woman's risk of developing breast cancer. The use of estrogen for women after menopause is currently also thought in general not to increase the risk of breast cancer, although there is some concern about its use for women who have other high-risk factors for developing the disease.

As was discussed in chapter VII, a subcutaneous mastectomy or a total mastectomy is sometimes requested as a preventive measure by women who are at very high risk of developing breast cancer. With subcutaneous mastectomy, some breast tissue is retained, so there is still some risk of developing breast cancer. Total mastectomy should almost completely eliminate the risk. However, a decision to have either of these operations clearly merits very careful consideration and counseling.

In this chapter I have addressed the issue of preventing breast cancer. It is our goal and will hopefully be a reality for many women. Clearly, there appear to be a number of steps we may take to reduce our risk of developing breast cancer. However, we are not yet able to prevent breast cancer for all women. Therefore, while keeping in sight our primary goal of preventing breast cancer, we must also attend to the secondary goal of preventing death from breast cancer. For those women for whom the disease is not preventable—millions worldwide, unfortunately—we must at least attempt to prevent death.

The way to do this is to get women involved in a program of breast-cancer screening from their early twenties on. All women must examine their breasts monthly (as outlined in chapter IV) from the time they are twenty years old. Periodic breast examinations should be done by a doctor. In addition, women should be involved in a screening mammography program as outlined by their physicians. The mammography should be performed on a machine that provides a low dose of radiation, since excessive radiation exposure itself has been shown to be carcinogenic. A properly performed mammographic examination done on a new, low-dose unit exposes a woman's breasts to a very small amount of radiation. The benefit of the screening mammography when done at appropriate intervals appears to outweigh its risks.

As a physician and as a woman, I believe that our primary goal must be to prevent breast cancer. There is certainly significant scientific information suggesting that modification of our life styles and dietary habits may help us achieve this goal. Meanwhile, we may offer many of those women for whom we are unable to prevent disease, prevention of death, the preservation of the breast, and a vastly improved outlook for their future.

CHAPTER XXI

Conclusion

As I wrote this book, I frequently had images of many women, both friends and patients of mine, who suffered needlessly and who died when they could have lived. I wrote out of love and concern for the hundreds of thousands of women who have suffered more than they needed to. I hope that this book will prevent future generations of women from unnecessary death and pain.

Breast cancer is so common an illness that it can be considered to occur in epidemic proportions. One of every eleven American women will develop the disease, and the number of women afflicted worldwide each year is astounding.

Although we continue to learn more about high-risk factors and prevention of the disease, any person with breasts is at risk of developing breast cancer. Even so, lives can be saved so easily.

Women who have a breast cancer diagnosed when it is still quite small, and before it has metastasized to the lymph nodes, have an excellent chance of being cured. And if it is diagnosed early enough, women can probably be offered the opportunity of being treated without having the breast removed and with excellent cosmetic results. If they do have a mastectomy, women whose lesions were diagnosed early are often better candidates for breast reconstruction and certainly are more likely to be cured.

We women must help ourselves. We must perform monthly breast self-examination. If we delay and deny when we do feel a lump, we are being our own worst enemies instead of our own best friends.

Women must learn and believe that tumors found when they are small are usually curable and can be treated with excellent cosmetic results. Armed with this knowledge, women must get involved in monthly self-screening, as well as being screened at appropriate intervals by their doctors and with mammography. We must keep ourselves healthy and we must encourage one another to stay healthy.

It seems to me that knowing the benefits of screening for the early detection of breast cancer should be a very powerful incentive for women. Once you believe it and are following the guidelines, share the information with your friends. There is no need for any of us to be haunted by the memories of suffering and illness that could so easily have been prevented.

Index